Would you like to live everyday without cravings, mood swings, energy lows and pain highs, while reducing your risks of acquiring one or more of the modern diseases like diabetes or heart disease? We will give you the tools to do just that with a very simple lifestyle that you can get excited about.

Have a better life with good tasting meals, desserts and snacks the whole family can enjoy.

Yummidy!

Yummidy!

A Low Carb Guide
and Meatless Cook Book

David M. Kennedy, CN
Sherry L. Laney

iUniverse, Inc.
New York Lincoln Shanghai

Yummidy!
A Low Carb Guide and Meatless Cook Book

iUniverse books may be ordered through booksellers or by contacting:

iUniverse
2021 Pine Lake Road, Suite 100
Lincoln, NE 68512
www.iuniverse.com
1-800-Authors (1-800-288-4677)

The information provided in this book is from the authors' experience and is not intended to replace the advice of your health care professional. Consult with your physician before starting any nutrition or exercise program especially if you are using prescription medications.

ISBN-13: 978-0-595-35985-1 (pbk)
ISBN-13: 978-0-595-80435-1 (ebk)
ISBN-10: 0-595-35985-X (pbk)
ISBN-10: 0-595-80435-7 (ebk)

Printed in the United States of America

Dedicated to those who think they can't

CONTENTS

Introduction

This book is for anyone who wants to make positive, healthy changes for themselves or for their family. It provides dozens of low carb recipes for entrees, side dishes, snacks, and desserts. It will help you to grasp concepts and to reaffirm ideas that will better your chances for long term success with the low carb lifestyle. You will become more aware of what you are eating and what happens when you eat it.

Why Low Carbohydrate? An aversion to fat, availability of increasingly simple carbs with increasingly sedentary lifestyles has been a health disaster in the US. Huge numbers of us are overweight and/or are suffering from the self inflicted modern ailments like heart disease and adult onset diabetes. The addiction to sugars and starches is widespread yet often unrecognized.

Most people that are on or have tried a low carb lifestyle do so because of weight concerns, and this is a major benefit, but there are other reasons including:

- Maintaining energy levels
- Appetite control
- Eliminating hypoglycemia
- Anti inflammatory
- Anti aging
- Reducing joint and muscle pain
- Reducing night sweats and hot flashes
- Reducing PMS symptoms
- Improving depression and anxiety
- Reducing or eliminating acid reflux and healing ulcers
- Reducing headache severity and frequency
- Reducing cholesterol and triglycerides
- Reducing blood pressure
- Reversing Atherosclerosis
- Reducing risk of stroke and heart attack
- Reversing Diabetes
- Reversing impotence
- Reducing acrylamide intake
- Reducing cancer risks

- Candida elimination diet
- Polycystic Ovary Syndrome
- Psoriasis
- Stress management

These conditions can all be impacted by the resulting weight loss, reduced inflammation, reduced insulin levels, and blood sugar control.

Why meatless? An alternative, more options, variety, choice. Those who already have a low carb lifestyle will expand their menus. Some may like the idea of a 'not bacon' diet or to finally be able to combine the benefits of low carb and meatless and try it for the first time. It can offer a low carb lifestyle for vegetarians who may take another look at where their diet is and where it is taking them.

We are going to provide you with a simple explanation of the Low Carbohydrate Lifestyle with a meatless alternative and describe the benefits of insulin and inflammation control.

Understanding low carb concepts

What are carbohydrates? Carbohydrates are compounds of carbon, oxygen, and hydrogen arranged as monosaccharides or multiples of monosaccharides. More simply put, sugars, starches, and fiber. Foods that can be high in carbohydrates include grains, foods made from grains (like bread, cereal, pasta), milk, most beans, most fruits, some vegetables, and all the foods that have added sugars like soda, candy and desserts. The other constituents of food are protein and fat.

Take a look at carbohydrate digestion. It begins in the mouth where an enzyme (amylase) starts breaking down starches into simpler sugars. Carbohydrate digestion actually slows when the food hits the stomach and starts up again when it enters the small intestine where additional enzymes continue the process. Most of the carbohydrate digestion occurs in the small intestine with the end product being glucose, fructose and galactose. These simple sugars are absorbed into the bloodstream and pass through the liver which converts the fructose and galactose into glucose. Glucose is used to fuel most of the bodies cells. Once inside the cell, enzymes break down the glucose into smaller fragments which get broken down further yielding the energy.

The liver stores and releases glucose as needed. During times of excess glucose, the liver converts that excess into glycogen which it stores in itself or in the muscles. During periods of low glucose the glycogen is converted back into glucose. The body has a limited capacity to store glucose as glycogen and when the glycogen is used up and glucose becomes unavailable the body turns to fat and protein to meet its energy needs.

It's important to understand how the glucose gets into the cells of our body. After we eat a food that contains enough starch or sugar, and glucose enters the blood stream, islets on the pancreas produce insulin which stimulates receptors on our cells which allow glucose to pass into the cell. This process provides fuel for the cells and keeps blood sugar from being too high.

Insulin is a powerful hormone that, when released, starts glucose utilization, stops fat burning and triggers fat storage. Overproduction of insulin has a definite link to most of the problems associated with a high carb lifestyle. There are several causes for the overproduction of insulin including:

- Intake of too many carbs relative to the amount of protein, fat and fiber in the meal
- Under eating or skipping meals
- Excessive caffeine use
- Elevated stress levels

All carbohydrates are not created equally and we can quantify their relative ability to affect blood glucose and insulin levels using the glycemic index. Higher glycemic foods will impact blood sugar levels, insulin production and inflammation more than low glycemic foods. An example of a high glycemic food is pasta, and an example of a low glycemic food is broccoli. One quarter cup of cooked pasta has the same ability to raise your insulin levels as nine cups of broccoli. Bread is considered a high glycemic food but whole wheat bread has a lower glycemic index than white bread due to the fiber that slows down digestion and absorption of carbohydrates slowing the rise of blood sugar. It's important to know that the amount of fat and protein in a meal also affects insulin production and that low glycemic foods are more easily counteracted and that high glycemic foods can be hard to counteract (if not impossible).

Here are some examples. If you have a piece of whole wheat toast, your insulin levels will rise (though not as dramatically as with white toast). If you eat the same piece of whole wheat toast with a three egg cheese omelette your insulin levels will likely stay flat thanks to the sufficient fat and protein. Of course, if you eat the same cheese omelette without toast there are no carbs and your insulin levels stay flat. If you eat that omelette with toast, home fries, and orange juice there is so much starch and sugar your insulin levels rise sharply. This is the meal to be most concerned with. Insulin tells your body to stop burning fat and to start storing fat and the rise in insulin will efficiently store the available saturated fats from the eggs and cheese. This is not to say that fat makes you fat. Your body will readily convert carbohydrates into fat when enough insulin is produced. It is more efficient however, to store available fat than to convert carbs into fat when insulin is released. Fat in your meal helps control the glycemic effect of carbs helping to control blood sugar levels. Fat will also make you feel more satisfied. Intake of fat is important as an energy source, in maintaining Omega 3 levels, and for hormone production.

# Glycemic Index
Glucose=100

Food	Value	Note
Grains		
Barley	25	2
Buckwheat	56	3
Bulgur	48	3
Rice, brown	55	3
Rice, instant	91	3
Millet	71	3
Cornmeal	68	3
Buckwheat	54	3
Cereal		
Quick Oatmeal	66	3
Steel Cut Oats	42	3
Puffed Wheat	74	3
Shredded Wheat	68	3
Muesli	66	3
Grape nuts	67	3
Rice Chex	89	3
All Bran	46	3
Corn Flakes	83	3
Cheerios	74	3
Cream of Wheat	66	3
Special K	54	3
Rice Crispies	82	3
Life	66	3
Breads		
Blueberry Muffins	59	3
Bagel plain	72	3
Pumpernickel	49	3
White	70	3
Rye	64	3
Pita	57	3

Crackers

Graham	74	3
Saltine	72	3
Rice cakes	80	3
Wheat thins	67	3

Pasta

Whole Wheat Pasta	45	3
Spaghetti	41	3
Linguine	46	3
Corn Pasta	78	3
Rice Pasta	92	3

Beans

Black	30	3
Garbanzo	34	3
Red lentils	27	3
Kidney	52	3
Lima	32	3
Pinto	39	3
Soy	16	2

Nuts

Cashews	22	2
Peanuts	14	2

Fruit

Apple	38	3
Apricot	57	3
Banana	52	3
Blueberry	30	2
Cantaloupe	65	3
Cherries	22	2
Dates	103	3
Fig	35	3
Dried Fig	80	3
Grapefruit	25	2
Grapes	46	3
Kiwi	58	3
Mango	51	3

Orange	43	3
Papaya	58	3
Peach	42	3
Pear	38	3
Pineapple	66	3
Plum	39	3
Raisins	60	3
Raspberry	32	2
Strawberries	32	2
Watermelon	72	3

Vegetables

Asparagus	<15	1
Broccoli	<15	1
Cabbage	10	1
Cauliflower	<15	1
Celery	10	1
Cucumber	<15	1
Eggplant	<15	1
Green Beans	<15	1
Lettuce	10	1
Mushroom	10	1
Onion	10	1
Peppers	<15	1
Spinach	<15	1
Zucchini	<15	1
Beets	64	3
Raw Carrot	47	3
Cooked Carrots	71	3
Green Peas	48	3
Sweet Corn	55	3
Sweet Potato	54	3
Baked Potato	85	3
French Fries	75	3
Instant Mash Potato	86	3
Tomato	15	1

Snacks

Corn Chips	68	3
Fruit Leather	99	3
Graham Cracker	74	3
Ice Cream Premium	38	3
Ice Cream Low Fat	43	3
Jelly Beans	80	3
Pop Corn	60	3
Potato Chips	57	3
Power Bar Chocolate	56	3
Pretzels	82	3

Drinks

Apple Juice	40	3
Beer	73	3
Carrot Juice	43	3
Coca Cola	63	3
Whole Milk	30	3
Skim Milk	46	3
Orange Juice	60	3
Pineapple Juice	46	3

Note
1-Use regularly in controlled portions with sufficient fat and protein
2-Use sparingly in controlled portions with sufficient fat and protein
3-Avoid

So What's the Problem?

Inflammation

Imagine the body healing a scrape or a brush burn. There is inflammation at the site as the body's immune system fights infection, the cells in the affected area are signaled to multiply, and new blood vessels form to nourish the new tissue, resulting in redness and swelling. The same thing happens inside our body when it is damaged by exposure to elevated levels of sugar. A constant intake of excessive carbs leads to a constant elevation of inflammation levels. The inflammation itself leads to the formation of more inflammatory substances sustaining the levels.

For many, the noticeable effect of elevated inflammation levels is increased muscle and joint pain, or 'waking up stiff and sore'. This can be due to eating too many carbs at one time causing rapidly increasing blood sugar levels.

Inflammation can be measured by C-Reactive Protein (CRP) levels. CRP is not found in food but is produced within the body and levels are strongly influenced by diet.

Chronic inflammation has been linked to many of our modern health problems especially atherosclerosis, heart attack, stroke, diabetes, cancer and Alzheimer's. Studies have shown that men and women who have chronic inflammation have a 66% greater risk of cognitive problems. Those with high CRP levels are twice as likely to develop colon cancer.

Excessive blood sugar and inflammation cause damage to artery walls and the body reacts to the damage by producing excess cholesterol to repair the damage and by generating an excess of cells on the artery wall. Healthy arteries are smooth and damaged arteries are thick and plaque covered. Excessive inflammation can cause a rupture of the plaque and a blockage downstream results, reducing or stopping blood flow to tissues and organs. Heart attacks and strokes can be caused by these blockages.

C-Reactive Protein is produced in large quantities by adipose (fat) cells especially those around the body's mid section (tummy area). The high output of CRP by fat cells make obesity a primary risk factor for atherosclerosis. Elevated inflammation levels are thought to interfere with the ability of glucose to enter the cell thereby contributing to diabetic conditions. The resulting elevated blood sugar levels cause additional cell and artery damage and increase CRP levels even further. Weight loss results in reduced CRP production thereby reducing inflammation levels. Lower inflammation levels lead to less artery damage and improved sugar utilization.

Studies have shown that subjects who ate high glycemic carbs such as potatoes, breakfast cereals, white bread, muffins and white rice had very high CRP levels and those who ate these foods and were overweight had the highest and most dangerous levels. Those with the highest CRP levels have five times the risk of developing cardiovascular disease and seven times the risk of having a stroke or heart attack.

Elevated blood sugar levels also result in the formation of excessive Advanced Glycation End Products (AGE's). AGE's are the end result of chemical reaction where proteins and DNA are damaged by exposure to sugar. Glycation chemistry is evident when food is 'browned' (ie bread to toast). This browning is occurring in the cells of the body through our entire life and is a major part of the aging process. Excessive amounts of sugar in the blood increase the rate and degree of damage. Nerve cells, cells in the retina of the eye and glomeruli of the kidney are very prone to glycation damage due to the higher glucose levels they receive explaining the additional risk for blindness, kidney disease and neuropathy in diabetics. Diabetics suffer an accelerated aging due to chronically high blood sugar. Studies have shown that traditional vegetarians have higher AGE levels than omnivorous groups mainly due to higher fructose intake. AGE's also increase inflammation levels throughout the body and contribute to reduced sugar utilization and higher blood sugar levels and therefore more AGE's.

Storing Fat

Our body anticipates more incoming carbs as we eat. For example, if you're eating a bagel, the body doesn't know that you are going to eat one bagel. It anticipates a second or third bagel and produces an excess of insulin as you eat. After the insulin reacts with the introduced sugar in the blood, the excess insulin continues to reduce the remaining blood sugar making us feel tired, craving a sweet or starch, and even degrading our mood. Insulin tells the body to utilize glucose, stop burning fat, and start storing fat. Chronically elevated insulin causes overproduction of cholesterol. It contributes to the desensitizing of the cells to insulin which leads to higher blood sugar levels and higher insulin demand and production. This excess insulin continues to signal fat storage and leads to higher CRP levels.

We have been given remarkable gifts that make our bodies very able to help keep us alive. We are hard wired to seek out glucose sources in sugars and starches. It's very natural to want them. When they are available we eat them. In most of the natural world, availability of carbs is seasonal. Winter/summer, wet season/dry season, there are times when carbs are plentiful and there are times when they are not available. The interesting fact is that one's ability to store fat during times of plenty helps them survive times without. When sugars and starches become available we are driven to eat them as part of the process to enhance our survival prospects. We eat the available sugar and starches causing our insulin levels to rise, stopping fat burning and starting fat storage. Excess insulin forces down our blood sugar and we are hungry again. Eating while the eating is good, storing fat while the sugar is available. When winter (or dry season) comes and carbs become scarce, insulin stays flat and we burn fat for energy, consuming low carb foods as we find them but still always seeking the glucose sources.

Many assume that skipping meals or eating less can help control weight and cholesterol levels but the body monitors how often you eat and how much you eat. If you decide to skip a meal or eat less than you need, your body thinks there is a shortage of food and that there is a danger of starvation. The next time you eat, your body tries to capture as much of the meal or snack as possible and store it as fat. It does that by releasing a high amount of insulin, which stops fat burning, starts fat storage, and drives down blood sugar levels with the excess insulin that is released. The drop in blood sugar increases the cravings for more carbs.

The ability to store fat has always been essential for survival and a very positive trait. Those that had the ability to store were more likely to survive lean times. In modern America with our modern food supply, this trait has become a liability as most live in the perpetual summer/wet season where there is a constant supply of carbs with no winter/dry season to burn off stored fat. The production of insulin to excessive levels day after day, month after month, year after year is abusing the gifts that we have been given and we are paying the price. The dramatic rise in obesity among adults and children in the US is staggering. Heart disease is this country's number one killer. Diabetes rates are skyrocketing. Fatigue, depression, mood swings and arthritis pain are common complaints. Again, all related to sugars, starches, and elevated inflammation and insulin levels.

Do you know how heavy and bulky a pound of butter is? That's what one pound of fat looks like and feels like. Now imagine twenty pounds, or forty. Have you ever felt how heavy twenty pounds is? Is that what you're carrying around with you all day? What a strain on your body. What a burden on your joints. Painful knees and feet can be a direct result of osteoarthritis caused by excess weight damage to joints.

Cholesterol

Cholesterol circulates in the blood mostly in the form of particles consisting of protein, fat and cholesterol. LDL cholesterol or low density lipoprotein is the main transporter of cholesterol in the blood stream from the liver to the cells.

LDL seems to encourage deposition of cholesterol in the arteries. HDL cholesterol or high density lipoprotein is known as the good cholesterol because it carries cholesterol away from the cells back to the liver where it is broken down and eliminated. Cholesterol is required by the body and is vital for proper brain and nerve function and to the production of Vitamin D, bile, sex hormones, and adrenal hormones. It is a structural component of cell membranes and also a vital repair mechanism for damaged arteries. Our liver is constantly producing cholesterol to meet our bodies needs.

Eating animal products, including eggs and dairy, can add to our total cholesterol level. About 15% of our blood cholesterol can come from the dietary sources. Eggs and dairy can be a good source of protein but if cholesterol is a concern there are some things to consider. Cutting the number of egg yolks and replacing with more egg whites, using Egg Beaters®, or replacing butter with Smart Balance® can help.

Food Cholesterol Content

Food	*Serving*	*Cholesterol (mg)*
Egg	One (50g)	210
Egg Yolk	One	210
Egg White	One	0
Egg Beaters	61g	0
Duck Egg	One	619
Cow Brain	100g	2054
Chicken Breast	100g	39
Beef	100g	65
Vegetable Oil	100g	0
Lean Fish	100g	45
Cream	100g	140
Cheese	100g	100
Butter	100g	260
Smart Balance	14g	0
Ice Cream	100g	45
Milk	100g	13
Vegetables, Fruit, Grains, Beans		0

Inflammation and excess insulin have many effects including raising our cholesterol levels. The constant elevation of insulin and inflammation caused by the constant intake of excess carbs over long periods of time causes an overproduction of cholesterol. The elevated insulin level is directing the body to store fat, combining with the inflammatory condition and with the over production of cholesterol, promoting plaque buildup. This 'clogging' of arteries can lead to reduced blood flow, high blood pressure, stroke, heart attack, Alzheimer's and impotence.

Reducing carb intake, eating regularly, and the subsequent reduction of insulin and inflammation levels allows the liver to stop overproducing cholesterol and levels can return to more normal. Modern cholesterol reducing drugs have a slight anti-inflammatory affect and impair the liver's cholesterol production.

Stress

An elevated stress level activates our sympathetic nervous system causing the release of many chemicals in our body including Cortisol which can damage our artery walls. Cortisol also causes an increase of glucose in the blood (itself increasing inflammation and AGE's) resulting in the release of insulin. The greater the stress, the greater the response inevitably leading to low blood sugar. The sympathetic system prepares our body for a fight or to take flight and another result is the constriction of blood vessels which raises blood pressure. High blood pressure also causes increased inflammation and artery damage. A properly done low carb lifestyle can help stress management by helping to keep blood sugar levels constant and allowing for better and more stable moods. Adequate protein intake helps assure proper neurotransmitter formation and helps control depression.

Diabetes

Type Two Diabetes, also known as Adult Onset Diabetes, is caused by the desensitizing of our cells receptors to insulin due to the regular high levels of insulin and chronic inflammation. Ironically, the pancreas must produce increasing amounts of insulin to overcome this as blood sugar levels continue to rise above normal. This condition is most often associated with excess body weight as fat cells themselves produce large amounts of C Reactive Protein and weight reduction often reverses or eliminates it.

Oxidants

Oxidants from pesticides in food, pollution, cigarette smoke, CRT radiation (TV's and monitors), enter the blood stream and cause damage to the arteries. They also alter LDL cholesterol. The resulting oxidized LDL cholesterol also causes damage to the artery walls and increases inflammation. Maintaining adequate antioxidant levels (ie Vitamins C and E) in the body not only has a direct beneficial effect on inflammation levels but protects cells and LDL cholesterol from damage.

Acid Reflux

So many low fat, high carb dieters suffer from Acid Reflux. High carb/lowfat life styles have many meals which are very low in protein. During each meal your body is expecting protein to be included and provides stomach acid for the start of its digestion. Without the protein to utilize the acid, the high acid levels cause damage to the upper digestive tract over time. Reflux and ulcers can be worsened by this excess acid. A steady routine of low carb meals that include protein will improve reflux and ulcers. Low carb meals can also help reduce intestinal gas.

So why can't I stop eating?

Reducing carb intake and maintaining proper weight is necessary, so why can't I stop eating? A brain scan study using normal hungry people showed that particular areas of their brain became active when they saw and smelled their favorite foods. These areas are the same to become active in cocaine addicts when they think about their next use. So, when it comes to cookies, this will help explain why 'one is too many and ten is not enough'.

We are hard wired to want carbs. It's part of who we are. Combine this with a readily available supply and a fat free society that promotes their benefits and we're set up for a fall.

Eating simple or complex carbs without enough fat, protein or fiber will cause a spike in insulin levels. This excess insulin forces down our blood sugar levels. The up shot of insulin and the subsequent fall in blood sugar creates a craving. Your brain wants a blood sugar spike and it will do what it has to do to get it. In addition to the craving, your mind will justify any action to get what it wants. It will tell you, 'You're not as fat as so and so', 'You won't get diabetes, someone else will', 'Low carb is really bad for you', 'What else do I have', 'I like to eat', 'Life without my favorite foods isn't worth living', 'Just this once'.

If you know someone who suffers from a more recognized addiction to tobacco or alcohol, you've probably heard the same excuses from them. The addicted brain is very powerful and you must do things right to beat it. With carb addiction, it's most important to control your blood sugar. Dramatic ups and downs in blood sugar levels cause mood swings, low energy, and cravings. Not a good place to be when fighting any addiction.

I have known many who, when they had decided things were bad enough, tried to get their health back by switching to a low fat diet. They start with rice cakes, dry toast, popcorn, skipping meals, etc., and what happens? Their blood sugar goes up, insulin goes up, the excess insulin produced forces down blood sugar causing cravings. Many are strong willed. Where one might last days or weeks, others fight on for months at a time, white knuckled, sweating, crying, until they finally break. Inevitably, they just couldn't take it anymore.

To succeed, you must work with who you are. You must understand the addiction. You can't let your brain talk you out of it. Any thing less will intensify the fight and increase the odds for failure. Give your self enough worth to pay attention to how you feel throughout the day. You will know when you are doing things right and when you are doing things wrong. It feels a lot better when you're doing things right. When you make a mistake, you will feel tired and have cravings. Think back to what went in your mouth about one to one and a half hours prior. If you look objectively, you can analyze the meal or snack to see what caused the increase in insulin and the subsequent drop in blood sugar. In doing so you will realize your mistake and it will reinforce what you have learned. If the meal or snack truly is a balanced/low carb one, and there is nothing to blame the negative effects on, then you probably under ate at your previous meal, skipped a meal, or waited too long to eat since your last meal.

No doubt, the first week of your new lifestyle will be tough and I recommend eating your way through it. Eat low carb choices all day if you have to. You will find the blood sugar leveling off, the cravings subsiding and you will enter a stable pattern. Then, it's important to stay in a routine of Breakfast, Snack, Lunch, Snack, Dinner, Snack, to satisfy all mechanisms and protect yourself from letdowns and weakness.

So many people say they can't eat breakfast and haven't for years. This is something we have taught ourselves to do without even realizing it. Look at modern breakfast foods, toast, bagels, cereal, juice, all high glycemic carbs. Eating like foods causes insulin levels to rise in excess and force down our blood sugar levels leaving us tired and craving. Most say that they are hungry an hour after they eat these breakfast foods. We slowly learn that it is less painful to not eat than to go through the low blood sugar episodes.

But look at what we've chosen instead. We don't eat until lunch or later. Our body thinks there is a food shortage and that we are starving. We stop burning fat. No matter what food we eat next, even a perfect low carb meal, our insulin levels will rise as our body does its thing keeping us alive, maintaining and storing fat. The excess insulin forces down the blood sugar making us crave sugars and starch which we either give in to or suffer though. Satisfying the craving with sugar or starch, we bring blood sugar and insulin levels up with the eventual excess insulin caused blood sugar drop. And so it goes through the rest of the day until bedtime and the next day we wake up groggy, perhaps with stiffness and elevated pain levels. The amount of sugar and starch before bedtime will explain why some days are better than others when you wake up. The more sugar and starch, the greater the inflammation levels and the greater the pain and stiffness, the harder it is to wake up, and we'll wake up with a poor mood (on the wrong side of the bed), etc..

When you start eating breakfast again in the low carb lifestyle you will realize the benefits. Better energy, better concentration, and no cravings. Remember, it's natural to be hungry, but hunger is different from cravings. Hunger tells you when to eat. Cravings tell you when to eat and what to eat.

Where am I now

There are several parameters which will give you an idea of how you are doing.

BMI   The Body Mass Index is being used to determine under, normal, and over weight. Calculate your BMI with the formula below:

BMI = weight(in pounds) x 705/height (in inches) squared
Or
BMI = weight(in kilograms)/height (in meters) squared

BMI	<18.5	Underweight
BMI	18.5–24.9	Normal
BMI	25–29.9	Overweight
BMI	>30.0	Obese

Cholesterol-desired results

Total	<200mg/dl
HDL	>40mg/dl
LDL	<130mg/dl
Total/HDL ratio <5.0	

Triglycerides

Normal	<150mg/dl
Borderline high	150–199mg/dl
High	200–499mg/dl
Very High	500+

Blood Pressure   Pressure in the arteries with the heart in compression is the systolic pressure (top number). Pressure in the arteries when the heart is relaxed is the diastolic pressure (bottom number).

140/90 is borderline high. If systolic pressure is above 140 or if diastolic pressure is above 90, blood pressure is considered high.

Blood Sugar   Glucose in the blood

65–109mg/dl normal

CRP   C-Reactive Protein
<1 mg/l Low risk
1–3 mg/l Moderate risk
>3mg/l High risk

Should I Change

Where are you on the 'Health Elevator' and are you going Up or Down? The trip going down: you've gained a few pounds, not as active, no energy, hypoglycemic, acid reflux, mood swings, uncomfortable muscle and joint pain, high cholesterol, high triglycerides, stressed, obese, headaches, ulcers, high blood pressure, diabetes, fibromyalgia, arthritis pain, depression, impotent, diagnosed atherosclerosis, morbidly obese, cancer, cardiac episode, disability, early death? Where do *you* want the elevator to stop? When you are on the way down things keep getting worse.

Change direction before it's too late and start back up to good health. You will feel better, enjoy your life more, and live longer. You have to do it for yourself but look at those whose lives you touch and what it will mean to them.

Making it happen

Insulin control and reduced inflammation from a low carb lifestyle is the cornerstone of feeling good and reducing the risks of disease and debilitation. Exercise is another important component. I have seen time and again the person who has decided things have gotten bad enough that they need to change. They start their low fat diet and join a gym. They work hard and deprive themselves of food they're used to eating. Two weeks latter they haven't lost weight, they get frustrated and give up. Why? Because they were eating a fat free bagel with juice or a banana before going to workout, which caused insulin to rise forcing the body to burn glucose for fuel and not burn fat. On the other hand, I have seen so many start low carb, see results within weeks, get excited, and then join a gym, accelerating their results. Results are very motivating whether it be weight loss, less pain, better moods, or lower cholesterol.

You don't have to join a gym to exercise. Something as simple as walking is a great way to improve your health and sense of well being. Exercise can speed up weight loss. It can reduce cholesterol and triglycerides, increase insulin sensitivity, improve blood flow and heart function and reduce blood pressure. Exercise will increase your endurance and make you stronger helping you perform everyday activities better. Perhaps most importantly, exercise can improve mood, decrease stress and the sympathetic response, reduce anxiety and depression, all of which strengthen motivation and addiction management.

Although you can consider any exercise beneficial, that with sufficient intensity will have the greatest benefit. One way to measure intensity is by calculating the target heart rate which is 60–90% of your maximum heart rate. When you are walking or exercising, your heart rate should be within the target range. If your heart rate is below the bottom number of the target heart rate you could be exercising harder. If your heart rate is above the top number you probably should reduce your pace. To calculate maximum heart rate (MHR) subtract your age from 220. Multiply the result by 0.6 and 0.9 to find the target heart rate (THR). For example, if you're 45 years old:

$$\text{MHR} = 220 - 45 = 175 \text{ beats per minute (bpm)}$$
$$175 \times 0.6 = 105 \text{ bpm}$$
$$175 \times 0.9 = 158 \text{ bpm}$$
$$\text{THR} = 105 \text{ to } 158 \text{ bpm}$$

Even minutes of exercise spread across the day will magnify results. Take your dog for a walk (even if you don't have one). Be sure your health care provider is in agreement with your exercise plan.

Explore your need for emotional and spiritual healing. Yoga has become extremely popular and can help with stress and addiction management.

There are some basic ideas that can help with the addictive nature of carbs:

- Don't have old favorite high carb foods in the house. They will call to you in moments of weakness.

- Try to avoid the people, the places and the things that are likely to make you eat the foods you are trying to stay away from.

- Success requires work and your accepting responsibility. Living a low carb lifestyle is your best shot for keeping your blood sugar levels stable and minimizing cravings.

- If you have a slip, learn from it. Chances are you won't feel as good as you would like afterwards. Remembering that may help you avoid the next one.

Eating low carb versions of familiar foods can be a big help in adding variety but they may not have the same taste and texture of the foods you've been eating so be ready to compromise. The benefits will outweigh the differences. There are many foods on the market that are being sold as low carb that really aren't. They may be reduced carb but certainly are not low. Using low carb bread as an example, one that is three grams of net carbohydrates per slice is low carb and will add up to six grams in a sandwich. Using <u>nine grams</u> of net carbs per slice 'low carb' bread will yield eighteen grams in a sandwich. Be aware that just because the label says low carb it doesn't mean that it's so. Read the nutrition facts to be sure.

What are net carbs? Net carbs are the total carbohydrates minus the carbs that won't impact blood sugar levels. Nonimpact carbs include fiber. Fiber is a carbohydrate made from glucose but it is in a form that does not break down easily. Using the example of bread again, a slice with a total carb count of seven with four grams of fiber would have a net carb or impact carb count of three grams per slice. Many foods, especially 'low carb' nutrition bars and candies, contain glycerin and are sweetened with sugar alcohols (ie Maltitol) . These are not counted as impact carbs but it has been my experience that they can stall progress when used in high amounts. It would be better to eat a low carb bar than to skip a meal and cause imbalance, but even using one bar daily can hurt your progress.

High sugar alcohol sweetened foods can taste good and be a nice treat but watch out if the addicted brain kicks in and you eat more than you should. Many of us will suffer from excessive gas and diarrhea and it shouldn't take too many episodes before you become leery of them. Foods containing three or four grams of sugar alcohols per serving are more reasonable but watch your own reaction to see what you can tolerate.

Try to keep your net carb total under 50 grams per day. Spread them out through the day. Remember, we are trying to minimize carbs, we won't eliminate them. We want to choose our carbs efficiently and make sure they are eaten with fat and protein. If you are not seeing any progress toward your goals, tighten up on carb intake. If you are feeling tired or having cravings after meals you know your carb intake is too high.

If your carb intake gets low enough you will enter ketosis. This is where your body is using fat as its energy source without glucose. Fat is converted to ketone bodies and the accumulation of ketone bodies in the blood is known as ketosis. If you notice that you have buttery breath, you are probably in ketosis. You can use ketosis test strips which will show the level of ketones that you have.

We are trying to manage an addiction. Keeping ourselves robust is a great advantage. If we get worn down, stressed out, it isn't very likely we can succeed. One way to stay strong is to use supplements to insure we are getting a good amount of necessary nutrients. A good high potency multivitamin is a start. If needed, you can add additional supplements to the multi to reach the desired levels of key nutrients such as:

Chromium	100–200 mcg
Vitamin E	400–800 iu
Vitamin C	500–1000mg

In my opinion, the best stress management tool is adequate amounts of B vitamins. You should try to get 25mg each of B1, B2, B3, B5, B6, and 50mcg of B12 even if you consider your stress levels low. Additional B-complex providing 50mg (B-50) of each of the above mentioned B vitamins and additional B12 should be used as needed if stress levels are high. Switching to a low carb lifestyle in itself can be stressful adding to everyday stress so don't be afraid to take B-50 complex once or twice a day. Your body uses a lot of B vitamins when we are stressed, maintaining proper brain chemistry etc., and if we don't take in enough the stress will begin to take its toll affecting mood, outlook, composure, energy levels, increasing cravings, etc.. B vitamins are water soluble and your body will use what it needs and get rid of the rest. Make sure you have enough daily. You will notice the difference. If the B vitamins bother your stomach take them with a meal that contains protein (which won't be a problem while doing low carb). This should minimize stomach discomfort. Fat in your meal will enhance the uptake of vitamins E and D.

Vegetarians generally have lower iron and B12 intake. Menstruating women especially should be sure to supplement iron at a level of 10–18 mg per day. Iron bisglycinate is a good non constipating iron compound. Calcium and magnesium are important nutrients for many reasons including reducing blood pressure, preventing muscle cramps, heart health, reducing insomnia and nervousness. Women should consider 1000–1200mg of calcium and 500–600mg of magnesium daily and men 250–1000mg calcium and 125–500mg magnesium. Adequate blood calcium levels can help prevent bone loss (osteoporosis). Calcium citrate is a good calcium compound. Citrate is bulkier so you will have to take more tablets than with other calcium compounds but it is more absorbable.

A tablespoon of flaxseed oil daily will provide Omega 3 essential fatty acids which are anti-inflammatory, reduce blood pressure, lower cholesterol and triglyceride levels, and necessary for normal functioning of the brain. Every cell in the body needs essential fatty acids. Two tablespoons of ground flax meal has the equivalent of one tablespoon of flax oil. If you're new to either the oil or the meal, start at a fraction of the dose and increase the amount over time until desired amount is reached. Too much too soon may cause uncomfortable intestinal reactions.

The amino acid Tyrosine can be very helpful controlling sugar and starch cravings as well as improving mood and stimulating the metabolism. It can be very useful early in the switch to low carb but also during stressful periods as an accessory to your B-complex. 500–1000mg between each meal and snack (taken one hour before or after food) is my preferred dose. A formula for dose is, 50mg for each pound of body weight divided as described above. It can also be used as needed basis for mood and stress management. Do not use tyrosine if you have thyroid disease, melanoma, or are using any prescription medication for mood or depression. Take Tyrosine one hour away from food as protein may reduce its benefit.

Health and well being involves an intricate dance between the systems of the body and our own behavior. Real homeostasis is the alignment of these systems and proper habits on our part. In addition to correct food intake, we need to stay sufficiently hydrated and get adequate sleep. Doing so will allow the body to work efficiently and harmoniously. Failing any of these will keep the body out of balance and frustrate our efforts and progress.

Let's Eat

We are going to show you how to enjoy some familiar foods while keeping the carb content low. There will be some ingredient and preparation differences but you should quickly become accustomed to them. You will soon start to see meals and food combinations you will want to try. Your imagination and innovation will be a big part of your success so don't be afraid to experiment.

Not only can you take advantage of low carb but you can use low cholesterol alternatives. Butter can be replaced with Smart Balance® or similar. The number of egg yolks can be reduced using more egg whites or by using Egg Beaters®. Even some soy milks are low carb.

There are many new low carb products available. Some are low carb and some are not so low. Some taste good and some are not so good.

Here are some of our favorites:

Todd's 2 Carb® Bagels—a versatile food. Great for breakfast as an egg sandwich or with butter, low carb jam, or cream cheese. Good size and very satisfying, they have one net carb per half bagel. I usually double toast them or toast them on a griddle to crisp them up. If you like them, they can be a big part of your weekly menu. High in protein (19g/half bagel) and fiber, and in several flavors, they can be used in sandwiches or with a variety of hot toppings. This is where your imagination comes in handy but count the net carbs of <u>anything</u> you add to the bagel.

Atkins® Brand Bread—good taste and texture with three net carbs per slice. Toasted or not, very good for sandwiches, as a side, or for use in recipes. Several flavors, good shelf life (but don't be afraid to freeze and use as needed).

La Tortilla Factory® low carb tortilla—from breakfast burrito, to wraps, to pizzas, these 3 net carb tortillas can play an important part in your day. Mama Lupes's is another 3 carb brand. If you can't get these, you might find Cali-Wraps®. Although the net carb count is higher (8g), they are much bigger and a half tortilla can be used in a serving.

MiniCarb® (Eat Well, Be Well) Granola makes a great breakfast or snack. To wet the Granola there are Splenda® Sweetened low carb soy milks (like Soy Slender® by Hain 1g net carb/8 oz) or you can find unsweetened soy milk (Westsoy® Unsweetened 1g net carb/8 oz) to use as is or sweeten to taste with Splenda® or stevia. Cows milk comes in reduced carb or you can use cream or cream cut with water (ie 3 parts cream, two parts water and sweetened to taste with Splenda® or stevia).

Tofu can be a regular menu item as a good low carb (about 3 grams net carb in a half pound) protein source. Quorn® turkey roast and ground beef provide a non soy vegetarian protein with good taste and texture. 90 grams of Quorn®

turkey roast provides 15 grams of protein with 2 net carbs, and 85 grams of ground beef style Quorn® has 13 grams of protein with 4 net carbs.

Multigrain Cutlets® (1g net carb, 15g protein/serving) and FriChik® (2g net carb, 12g protein/serving) by Worthington, Boca Burgers (1g net carb, 13g protein/serving) and Quorn Naked Cutlets® (3g net carb, 11g protein) are examples of easy to use low carb vegetarian proteins that can simply be served with sides of low glycemic vegetables as a complete meal. Any can make a good sandwich. White Wave® Seitan (2g net carb, 31g protein) or Vegetarian Stir Fry Strips (2g net carb, 22g protein) can be used to make familiar dishes. Lightlife makes a variety of soy 'deli meats' and a hot dog substitute called Smart Dogs® (1g net carb, 9g protein per link). Yves Canadian Veggie Bacon is also handy to have around, very tasty and versatile, with 1 gram net carb and 17 grams of protein in three slices.

Black soy beans are the choice for bean recipes and Eden® brand canned has 1 gram of net carb and 11 grams of protein in a half cup serving. Good taste and texture.

Salads are popular as meals and can be a good choice. Be sure to watch the carb count of add ons, and be sure to have enough fat and protein with it. The salad dressing can add carbs and fat free varieties are more likely to have high carb counts. Homemade olive oil and vinegar dressing is good or there are several low carb brands available. Kraft Carb Well® (0 net carb), for example, comes in several flavors.

MiniCarb® (Eat Well, Be Well) Foods provides the mainstay of our baked good needs with several low carb high protein mixes. Most important are the 0 net carb Baking Mix and the 0 net carb Biscuit Mix. Some others are Pancake Mix, Bread Mix, and Chocolate Cake Mix. We use the baking mix to make an array of muffins which serve as a meal or a handy snack. It's also used to make several kinds of cookies and treats which can be used as a snack or a dessert. It also provides an assortment of biscuits (including some sweet) which can enhance a meal or be used as a meal, snack or dessert.

Low carb ice cream makes a nice evening snack. There are many national and local brands available. Find one you like that's three net carbs or less per serving and not too high in sugar alcohols (<6–7g per serving).

When using Peanut Butter, use brands that are 100% peanuts. Most of the major brands have sugar added to them.

One of the low carb chocolate chips we use are Russell Stover® Net Carb chocolate candy chips. 0.8 gram net carb per serving and 15.2 net carbs per 10 ounce bag. Carbsense makes a sugar alcohol free version which is higher in net carbs (3.8 per ounce).

We use Spectrum® brand Canola and Olive oils. They are cold pressed oils (verses solvent extracted) without solvent residues, and are of good quality.

Too much aspartame can cause fat burning to stop, so stevia and Splenda® are the preferred sweeteners. Aspartame is used to sweeten many commercial diet drinks. Water is a better choice but there are a variety of Splenda® sweetened drinks available. You can make several sweet drinks (hot or cold) using herbal teas (caffeine free) with stevia. We use Now Foods® brand liquid stevia extract.

You need to be aware that there is a difference between the Splenda® used in making commercial products and that sold for tabletop use. The following is an excerpt from an e-Mail I received from the makers of Splenda®:

"The caloric and carbohydrate content for SPLENDA(R) Brand Sweetener is as follows:
SPLENDA(R) Granular
1 tsp = 0.5 gm carb = 2 calories
one half cup = 12 gm carb = 48 calories
1 cup = 24 gm carb = 96 calories

*1 tsp. = 1 serving

Packet of SPLENDA
(R) 1 packet = .9 gm of carb = 4 calories

*1 packet has the sweetness of 2 tsp of sugar

Note: Per U.S. labeling laws, anything with less than 5 calories per serving, is properly labeled as "zero" or no-calorie."

"Note: The calories and carbohydrates in SPLENDA(R) No Calorie Sweetener come from dex-trose and/or maltodextrin, which are added for bulk. Sucralose, the sweetening ingredient in SPLENDA(R) Brand Sweetener, has no calories and is not a carbohydrate.

Granular—sucralose, maltodextrin (0.5 gram per serving) Packets—sucralose, maltodextrin and dextrose (less than 1 gram per packet)."

As noted, the Splenda® package is labeled 'No Calorie Sweetener' and the nutrition facts states calories 0 and Total Carb. less than 1 gram. Even though the serving size is 1 teaspoon, this gives the impression that there are no calories and therefore no carbs and no reason to limit its use. Wrong.

A recipe that calls for one cup of Splenda® will add 24 grams (net) of a carbo-hydrate that has a glycemic index higher than Jelly Beans, baked potato or instant rice. It must be used sparingly.

The majority of executives, engineers, dieticians, etc., that are responsible for making decisions on the products they produce are themselves addicted to sugars and really don't understand low carb reasoning. The same may be said for the author of a recent best selling book that claims to be a sensible alternative to the Atkins Diet. This book offers people (and the author) what they want to hear (and eat). These trusted sources help so many fail at trying to control their addictions and to eventually giving up. Staying within the program and cautiously avoiding "help" from these addicts that don't understand is essential. Remember they will offer some things that your own addiction is more than willing to accept.

The following are examples of our meal plans. They are just suggestions to give you some ideas so don't be afraid to mix them up and make them convenient. Add a small salad or a vegetable dish to any meal.

	Day 1	Day 2	Day 3
Breakfast	Bagel&Cream Cheese	Frittata with Toast	Granola
Snack	Flax Muffins	ChocolateChpCookie	Lemon Muffins
Lunch	Turkey Wrap	Pizza	Ham Sandwich
Snack	Brownie	Hazelnut Bar	Spice Cookies
Dinner	Vegetable Lasagna	Sesame Tofu & veg	Chili and Biscuits
Snack	Ice Cream & P Butter	PB Swirl Cake	Cheese Cake

	Day 4	Day 5	Day 6
Breakfast	Breakfast Burrito	Pancakes	French Toast
Snack	Maple Biscuit	Sour Cream Muffins	Cinnamon Biscuit
Lunch	Beans& Franks	Salad	Bean Enchilada
Snack	Crm Cheese Biscuit	Celery Soup	Strawberry Muffins
Dinner	Stuffed Zucchini	Tofu Stir Fry	Chicken&Pasta
Snack	Choco-Walnut Squares	Strawberry Tort	Root Beer Float

Day one of this menu starts out with a half bagel with cream cheese (2 net carb) for breakfast. Two flax muffins (3.2 net carb) for snack. A vege-turkey wrap with lettuce and mayo (5.0 net carb) for lunch. A brownie for afternoon snack (2.8 net carb). Vegetable lasagna (5.5 net carb) for dinner and Vanilla Ice Cream with peanut butter and chocolate chips for evening snack (4.7 net carb). Total net carb 23.3.

Day two of this menu starts out with a Frittata with Toast (5.3 net carb) for breakfast. Three Chocolate Chip Cookies (3.0 net carb) for morning snack. An eight slice tortilla pizza (9.6 net carb) for lunch. A Hazelnut Bar for afternoon snack (3.0 net carb). Sesame Tofu & green beans (7.0 net carb) for dinner and a slice of Peanut Butter Swirl Cake for evening snack (2.9 net carb). Total net carb 30.8.

Day three of this menu starts out with a simple bowl of low carb granola and low carb milk or soy milk (~5.0 net carb) for breakfast. Two Lemon Muffins (2.2 net carb) for morning snack. A vege-ham sandwich with lettuce and mustard (8.0 net carb) for lunch. Three Walnut Spice cookies for afternoon snack (2.4 net carb). Southwestern Chile and a biscuit (9.3 net carb) for dinner and a slice of Chocolate Almond Cheese Cake for evening snack (4.4 net carb). Total net carb 31.3.

Day four of this menu starts out with a Breakfast Burrito (5.0 net carb) for breakfast. Two Maple Biscuit (3.0 net carb) for morning snack. Beans& Franks (3.6 net carb) for lunch. Two Cream Cheese Biscuits for afternoon snack (3.8 net carb). Stuffed Zucchini (4.5 net carb) for dinner and a Chocolate Walnut Square for evening snack (3.8 net carb). Total net carb 23.7.

Day five of this menu starts out with 2 Pancakes with butter, low carb maple syrup, and whipped cream (1.3 net carb) for breakfast. Two Sour Cream Muffins (3.6 net carb) for morning snack. A salad with 2 cups of green leaf lettuce, cheese and/or baked tofu pieces, sliced olives, and dressing (3.0 net carb) for lunch. Celery Cream Soup for afternoon snack (3.2 net carb). Tofu Stir Fry (6.4 net carb) for dinner and a piece of Strawberry Tort for evening snack (3.9 net carb). Total net carb 21.4.

Day six of this menu starts out with 2 pieces of French Toast with butter and low carb maple syrup (6.6 net carb) for breakfast. Two Cinnamon Biscuits (2.4 net carb) for morning snack. A Bean Enchilada (6.1 net carb) for lunch. Two Strawberry Muffins for afternoon snack (1.0 net carb). Chicken, Spinach & Black Soybean Pasta (6.9 net carb) for dinner and a Root Beer Float for evening snack (3.0 net carb). Total net carb 27.0.

Make sure to include the net carbs of any add ons in your total. This doesn't include beverages so watch for added carbs from things that are such a normal part of your day that you don't even consider them, like half & half or sweetener in your tea or coffee. And yes, if you eat six cookies instead of three cookies, they count too.

The following recipes are going to give you some very good meals and snacks to get started with. More importantly, they're going to open the door to your ideas and some of your favorite recipes. Some of the ingredients and techniques may not be what you're used to but it won't take long to get familiar with them.

Remember, you can replace ingredients with those you are more comfortable with. Recipes calling for cream can use low carb soy milk or even water. Butter can be replaced with something like Smart Balance® or soy margarine. Egg yolks can be reduced by using more egg whites (one egg and six whites for 4 eggs) or eliminated with Egg Beaters® (one cup equals 4 eggs). Replacing ingredients will have effects on the finished product taste and texture so experiment and see what you like. Just keep in mind some of the basic principles like watching the carb count and glycemic index of ingredients and having enough fat and protein to slow down the carbs you use.

The recipes are in categories:
Breakfasts and Snacks
Entrees
Side Dishes
Desserts and more snacks

Use these categories as a guideline only. Mix them up to suit your taste and schedule but remember to eat breakfast and then eat regularly during the day.

Breakfast and Snacks

Maple Granola Biscuits

1 cup no carb bake or biscuit mix	0.0 gram net carb
1/4 cup no carb Maple Syrup	0.0 gram net carb
1/4 cup Splenda®	6.0 gram net carb
2 extra large eggs	0.5 gram net carb
1/3 cup water	0.0 gram net carb
1 teaspoon vanilla extract	0.5 gram net carb
1/3 cup vegetable oil	0.0 gram net carb
1/4 cup lo carb Granola	2.0 gram net carb
(or ¼ cup sliced almonds)	1.8 gram net carb

Combine ingredients in large bowl and stir until combined.

Spray oil or grease baking pan. Spoon batter on pan.

Bake 20 minutes in preheated 325 degree oven.

Cool. Lay biscuit flat on plate and cut horizontally. Spread half with cream cheese mix (to 6 tablespoons (3oz) cream cheese add a few drops of stevia liquid extract to taste, blend) or spread on top without cutting. Adds 0.4 gram net carb per biscuit. Adding a teaspoon of low carb jam will give some color and flavor to the cream cheese (0.1 grams net carb per biscuit).

Makes 6 Biscuits.   1.5 gram net carb each

Delicious!

Cinnamon Flax Muffins

1 cup MiniCarb® bake mix	0.0 gram net carb
½ cup ground flax seeds	4.9 gram net carb
1/4 cup Splenda	6.0 gram net carb
1 teaspoon Stevia Liquid Extract	0.0 gram net carb
1 teaspoon cinnamon	0.6 gram net carb
2 extra large eggs	0.8 gram net carb
3/4 cup water	0.0 gram net carb
(or ½ cup water + ¼ cup soy or low carb milk or cream)	(varies)
1 teaspoon vanilla extract	0.5 gram net carb
¼ cup vegetable oil	0.0 gram net carb

325 degree oven.

Combine MiniCarb® mix, flax seeds, Splenda® and cinnamon in large bowl.

Combine eggs, milk, water, vanilla, stevia and oil in medium bowl. Add to dry ingredients and stir until combined.

Spoon batter into muffin cups, no stick or greased muffin pan. Sprinkle with mixture of cinnamon and Splenda® if desired.

Bake 20 minutes.

Makes 8 muffins.   1.6 gram net carb each

Yummidy Yum!

Scrambled Eggs with Bread Cubes

1 slice low carb bread	3.0 gram net carb
2 tablespoons Butter	0.0 gram net carb
4–6 eggs	1.6–2.4 gram net carb

Cube 1 slice of low carb bread into ½ inch pieces.
Saute in 2 tablespoons of melted butter until browned.
Remove from pan.

Pour desired number of beaten eggs into pan and cook as you would scrambled eggs.

When eggs are almost done stir in bread crumbs.

Yield 2–3 servings   2.3–2.7 gram net carb each

You will be surprised by the flavor!

Blueberry Streusel Muffins

1 cup MiniCarb® bake mix	0.0 gram net carb
2 teaspoons liquid stevia extract	0.0 gram net carb
¼ teaspoon cinnamon	0.2 gram net carb
½ cup blueberries (fresh or frozen)	8.2 gram net carb
¼ cup vegetable oil	0.0 gram net carb
1 extra large egg	0.4 gram net carb
½ cup water	0.0 gram net carb
or low carb milk, soy milk	Varies
grated zest of half a lemon	0.3 gram net carb

Combine MiniCarb® and cinnamon in bowl.

In large bowl add egg then water, stevia, oil and lemon zest. Beat well.

Blend in dry ingredients; do not over mix. Stir in blueberries.

Spoon batter equally into muffin pan.

Sprinkle muffins with Splenda® and grated lemon zest mixture if desired.

Bake 20 minutes

Makes 6 muffins   1.5 gram net carb each

A Yummidy plus!

Spinach Frittata

1 tablespoon butter	0.0 gram net carb
4 extra large eggs	1.6 gram net carb
½ cup frozen spinach (thawed)	2.0 gram net carb
2 slices Swiss cheese diced	3.0 gram net carb

Place a 10 inch oven proof skillet on medium heat, melt butter and pour in beaten eggs, spinach, and cheese.

Cook without stirring for two minutes.

Place in 350 degree preheated oven and bake for five minutes.

Cut into 4 pieces   1.7 gram net carb each

Looks good, tastes good!

Zucchini Mushroom Frittata

6 extra large eggs	2.4 gram net carb
½ cup Swiss cheese diced	3.4 gram net carb
¼ cup water	0.0 gram net carb
½ teaspoon garlic powder	1.7 gram net carb
¼ teaspoon seasoned pepper	0.2 gram net carb
1 cup shredded zucchini	1.4 gram net carb
1 medium tomato chopped	3.3 gram net carb
1 cup sliced mushrooms	1.5 gram net carb

In medium bowl combine beaten eggs, cheese, water, and spices.

Spray a 10 inch oven proof skillet with oil. Over medium heat saute zucchini, tomato, and mushrooms until tender. Pour egg mixture into skillet, stirring well. Cover, cook over low heat for 15 minutes or until cooked on bottom and almost set on top. Remove lid and place under preheated broiler for 2–3 minutes

Cut into 6 pieces   2.3 gram net carb each

Yummidy morning, noon or night!

Orange Marmalade Muffins

1 cup MiniCarb® mix	0.0 gram net carb
2 tablespoons Splenda®	3.0 gram net carb
1 extra large egg	0.4 gram net carb
½ cup water	0.0 gram net carb
(or ½ cup soy, low carb milk or cream)	(varies)
¼ cup canola oil	0.0 gram net carb
½ teaspoons vanilla extract	0.0 gram net carb
grated zest of ½ lemon (approx 1 Tablespoon)	0.3 gram net carb
2 tablespoons low carb orange marmalade	2.0 gram net carb

350 degree oven

Combine MiniCarb® mix, Splenda® in large bowl. In medium bowl whisk egg, water, vanilla, oil and lemon zest. Pour liquid over dry ingredients and fold in with spatula until combined.

Fill muffin cups approx half full with batter. Place teaspoon of marmalade in each. Top with remaining batter. The marmalade does not have to be completely covered.

Sprinkle with additional Splenda® and lemon zest if you choose.

Bake 20 minutes.

Yield 6 muffins   1.0 gram net carb each

Yummidy, Orange.

Baked Eggs

8 eggs	3.2 gram net carb
4 cups Spinach leaf	1.6 gram net carb
¼ cup grated cheddar cheese	0.4 gram net carb
¼ cup cream	1.7 gram net carb
4 tablespoons butter	0.0 gram net carb
Salt and pepper	0.4 gram net carb

Bring a saucepan of water to a boil, add spinach leaves, and parboil for about one minute. Remove spinach from water, drain and rinse with cool water. Squeeze out excess water.

Preheat oven to 350

Using 4 ramekins, small souffle dishes or pyrex custard cups, rub each generously with butter. Divide the spinach between the 4 cups. Break two eggs into each cup. Salt and pepper to taste, add cheese and cream in equal amounts to each.

Place in oven. Bake until egg whites are just set (approximately ten minutes).

Turn out on to buttered low carb toast or a biscuit.

Makes 4 servings.   1.8 grams net carb each

Delicious!

Peanut Butter and Jelly Muffins

1 cup MiniCarb® bake mix	0.0 gram net carb
1 Teaspoon Stevia Liquid	0.0 gram net carb
1 extra large egg	0.4 gram net carb
¼ cup peanut butter (100% peanuts)	5.0 gram net carb
½ cup water	0.0 gram net carb
or low carb milk, soy milk, or cream	Varies
¼ cup vegetable oil	0.0 gram net carb
2 Tablespoons low carb fruit spread	4.0 gram net carb

350 degree preheated oven

Put MiniCarb® bake mix in a bowl. Combine egg, peanut butter, water, oil and stevia in a separate bowl. Blend until smooth. Pour liquid over bake mix and fold in with spatula until combined.

Fill muffin cups about half full with batter. Place one teaspoon of fruit spread in center of each. Top each muffin with remaining batter. Fruit spread does not need to be completely covered.

Sprinkle tops with a little bit of Splenda® if desired.

NOTE: For a variety use several kinds of fruit spread—blueberry, strawberry and raspberry have the strongest flavors.

If you choose to use Almond Butter the carb count is a little less than Peanut Butter.

Bake 20 minutes.

Makes 6 muffins   1.6 gram net carb each

Mmm mmm!

French Toast

4 slices low carb bread	12.0 gram net carb
1 tablespoon butter	0.0 gram net carb
2 extra large eggs	0.8 gram net carb
2–3 drops Almond extract	0.0 gram net carb
3 tablespoons water	0.0 gram net carb
or low carb milk, soy milk, or cream	Varies
¼ teaspoon cinnamon	0.2 gram net carb

Beat eggs, almond extract, Half and Half, and cinnamon together.

Melt butter in medium heat pan. Dip bread into egg mixture and press in to help bread absorb. Place wet slices on hot pan. Brown both sides.

Serve with butter, no carb maple syrup, and slivered almonds if desired.

Makes 4 pieces   3.3 grams net carb each

Great!

Chocolate Muffins

1 cup MiniCarb® bake mix	0.0 gram net carb
1/4 cup unsweetened cocoa powder	4.5 gram net carb
3 teaspoon stevia liquid extract	0.0 gram net carb
2 extra large egg	0.8 gram net carb
¾ cup water	0.0 gram net carb
or ½ cup low carb milk, soy milk and ¼ cup water	Varies
1/4 cup vegetable oil	0.0 gram net carb
½ teaspoons vanilla extract	0.0 gram net carb

325 degree oven

Combine MiniCarb® mix and cocoa in large bowl.

In medium bowl combine egg, water, oil, stevia and vanilla. Mix well until smooth.

Pour liquid over dry ingredients and fold with spatula until combined. Spoon batter equally into muffin cups and sprinkle each with a little Splenda® if desired.

Bake 20 minutes.

Makes 6 muffins   0.9 gram net carb each

These muffins taste like dessert!

Chocolate Sour Cream Muffins

¼ cup low carb chocolate chips	3.2 gram net carb
1 teaspoon butter	0.0 gram net carb

Melt chocolate on low heat with butter—set aside.

2 tablespoons softened butter	0.0 gram net carb
2 tablespoons Splenda®	3.0 gram net carb
1 extra large egg	0.4 gram net carb
¼ cup sour cream	4.0 gram net carb
1 teaspoon Stevia Liquid Extract	0.0 gram net carb
½ cup water	0.0 gram net carb
2 tablespoons vegetable oil	0.0 gram net carb
½ teaspoon vanilla extract	0.0 gram net carb
1 cup MiniCarb® bake mix	0.0 gram net carb

325 degree oven

In medium bowl beat softened butter and Splenda® with electric mixer (approx 2 minutes). Add egg, vanilla, stevia, water and sour cream. Beat until smooth. Fold into MiniCarb® mix until combined.
Pour melted chocolate mixture over batter and using a knife cut through batter several times to swirl chocolate.
Spoon equally into muffin cups.

Bake 20 minutes.

Makes 6 muffins   1.8 gram net carb each

Chocolidy

Breakfast Burrito

4 eggs	1.6 gram net carb
½ cups shredded cheese (cheddar, Monterey jack)	1.4 gram net carb
2 tablespoons cream cheese	0.8 gram net carb
dash cumin powder (to taste)	0.1 gram net carb
dash cayenne powder (to taste)	0.1 gram net carb
2 tortillas (low carb)	6 gram net carb

Spread one tablespoon of cream cheese down center of tortilla.

Scramble eggs in skillet adding cumin and cayenne. While cooking, push eggs into 2 equal log shapes that will fit into rolled tortilla. Place hot eggs in tortilla, add shredded cheese. Roll up tortilla. Folding in edge while rolling will help seal ends.
Using salsa will add ~ 1 gram net carb per tablespoon

Makes 2 servings   5.0 gram net carbs each using three net carb tortillas

Buenos dias!

Lemon Poppy Seed Muffins

1 cup low carb bake mix	0.0 gram net carb
2 teaspoons stevia liquid extract	0.0 gram net carb
2 tablespoons poppy seeds	2.2 gram net carb
1 extra large egg	0.4 gram net carb
½ cup water	0.0 gram net carb
or low carb milk, soy milk	Varies
¼ cup vegetable oil	0.0 gram net carb
grated zest of ½ lemon	0.3 gram net carb
3 tablespoons fresh lemon juice	3.9 gram net carb

350 degree oven.

Combine MiniCarb® mix, poppy seeds and lemon peel.

In medium bowl combine egg, water, stevia, oil and lemon juice. Stir into dry ingredients until just combined.

Spoon batter into muffin pan. Sprinkle each with Splenda® if desired.

Bake 20 minutes.

Makes 6 muffins.   1.1 gram net carb each

Enjoy!

Strawberry Muffins

1 cup MiniCarb® bake mix	0.0 gram net carb
2 teaspoons Liquid Stevia Extract	0.0 gram net carb
1 extra large egg	0.4 gram net carb
¾ cup water	0.0 gram net carb
or low carb milk, or soy milk	Varies
½ teaspoon vanilla extract	0.0 gram net carb
1 teaspoon lemon juice	0.3 gram net carb
¼ cup vegetable oil	0.0 gram net carb
4 large strawberries, chopped	2.0 gram net carb

325 degree preheated oven

Place MiniCarb® bake mix in large bowl.

In medium bowl beat egg, Stevia, water, vanilla and oil. Mix well. With spatula stir into baking mix until combined. Fold in strawberries.

Spoon equally into muffin pan.

Sprinkle each muffin with some Splenda® mixed with grated lemon zest if desired.

NOTE: These muffins are best eaten the same day. The baked strawberries tend to disappear as time goes by.

Bake 20 minutes.

Makes 6 muffins   0.5 gram net carb each

Absolutely delicious

Cinnamon Biscuits

1 cup lo carb biscuit or baking mix	0.0 gram net carb
¼ cup Splenda®	6.0 gram net carb
2 extra large eggs	0.8 gram net carb
4 tablespoons butter softened	0.0 gram net carb
⅔ cup water	0.0 gram net carb
or cream, low carb milk or soy milk	varies
⅓ cup oil	0.0 gram net carb
½ teaspoon vanilla extract	0.0 gram net carb
½ teaspoon cinnamon	0.4 gram net carb

350 degree oven

Combine all ingredients until moistened. Batter may still have some small lumps. Spoon batter in equal portions onto a greased baking sheet. Sprinkle each biscuit with a small amount of Splenda® and cinnamon if desired.

Bake 20 minutes or until golden brown.

Spread with butter or cream cheese if desired.

Makes 6 very large biscuits   1.2 gram net carb each

Wonderful!

Cream Cheese Biscuits

1 cup low carb biscuit mix or bake mix	0.0 gram net carb
⅓ cup Splenda®	8.0 gram net carb
2 extra large eggs	0.8 gram net carb
4 tablespoons butter softened	0.0 gram net carb
⅔ cup water	0.0 gram net carb
or low carb milk or soy milk	Varies
⅓ cup oil	0.0 gram net carb
½ teaspoon vanilla extract	0.0 gram net carb
3 tablespoons cream cheese softened	1.2 gram net carb
1 tablespoon Splenda®	1.5 gram net carb

Preheated 350 degree oven

Combine biscuit mix, Splenda®, eggs, butter, water, oil and vanilla in large bowl until just moistened. Batter may still have some small lumps. Spoon batter in 6 equal portions onto a greased cookie sheet.

In small bowl combine cream cheese and Splenda®, mixing until spreading consistency.

Spoon biscuit batter in equal portions onto a greased cookie sheet. Drop equal amounts of the cream cheese mixture into the middle of each biscuit. Sprinkle with a small amount of Splenda® if desired.

Bake 22 minutes or until golden brown.

Makes 6 very large biscuits   1.9 gram net carb each

Mmm, Mmm Yum!

Chocolate Coconut Almond Muffins

1 cup MiniCarb® bake mix	0.0 gram net carb
2 teaspoons stevia liquid extract	0.0 gram net carb
¼ cup unsweetened cocoa powder	4.5 gram net carb
1 extra large egg	0.4 gram net carb
1 cup water	0.0 gram net carb
or low carb milk, soy milk	Varies
¼ cup vegetable oil	0.0 gram net carb
¼ cup shredded coconut toasted	1.7 gram net carb
1 teaspoon almond extract	0.0 gram net carb
1 tablespoons sliced almonds	0.5 gram net carb

325 preheated degree oven.

Toast coconut on a baking sheet for about 2½ minutes. Be careful not to burn.

In a larger bowl combine MiniCarb® mix, cocoa powder and coconut.

In medium bowl combine egg, water, stevia, oil and almond extract. Stir into dry ingredients until just combined.

Spoon batter into muffin pan. Sprinkle each with sliced almonds and press into muffin top slightly.

Bake 20 minutes.
Makes 6 muffins.

1.2 gram net carb each

Enjoy!

Pancakes

½ cup low carb bake mix	0.0 gram net carb
1 extra large egg	0.4 gram net carb
1 tablespoon vegetable oil	0.0 gram net carb
½ cup water	0.0 gram net carb
few drops of vanilla extract	0.0 gram net carb

Combine all ingredients in a bowl and gently stir until all lumps are dissolved. Let stand for 2 minutes.

Heat lightly buttered griddle to 375 degrees. Pour approximately ½ the batter per pancake onto griddle. Cook about 2 minutes per side, turning pancakes only once.

Makes 4 thick pancakes.   0.2 gram net carb each

Variations:

top with:
butter
no carb syrup
Heavy cream whipped and flavored with vanilla and Splenda®
Sprinkle some ground walnuts on top of whipped cream.

Slice up a couple of strawberries and fold into batter before cooking. Blueberries are also a great choice.

These pancakes couldn't get any easier and the taste is pure heaven!

Shirred Eggs

4 eggs	1.6 gram net carb
4 teaspoons butter	0.0 gram net carb
Salt and pepper	0.4 gram net carb
2 slices low carb bread	6.0 gram net carb

Preheated 325 degree oven.

For each egg melt one teaspoon of butter in a ramekin or a muffin tin. Break an egg into the ramekin or muffin cup, salt and pepper to taste. Bake approximately 9 minutes or until eggs are set. Serve immediately with buttered low carb toast.

Makes 2 servings.   4.0 gram net carb each

Quick, easy and good!

Scrambled Eggs with Asparagus

4 stalks asparagus	1.3 gram net carb
½ tablespoon Butter	0.0 gram net carb
4 eggs	1.6 gram net carb
1 teaspoon shallot diced	0.6 gram net carb
¼ cup heavy cream	1.7 gram net carb
2 tablespoons Parmesan Cheese grated	0.4 gram net carb
⅛ teaspoon pepper	0.1 gram net carb

Cut asparagus into 1 inch pieces and steam until done but still firm. Add to scrambled eggs about 1 minute before the eggs are done cooking.
Saute the shallot in a small saucepan with butter (about 3 minutes).
Add cream and bring to a boil. Add cheese and pepper, stirring until cheese has melted. Remove from heat. Spoon over the eggs asparagus mixture.

Yield 2 servings   2.9 gram net carb each

Great use of the parmesan cheese sauce!

Tofu Scramble

8 ounces extra firm tofu (one half block)	2.5 gram net carb
¼ teaspoon tamari (soy sauce)	0.1 gram net carb
¼ teaspoon turmeric	0.9 gram net carb
¼ cup onion chopped	3.5 gram net carb
¼ teaspoon granulated garlic	0.4 gram net carb
2 tablespoon olive oil	0.0 gram net carb
Salt and pepper	0.4 gram net carb

Press excess water from the tofu and crumble to an even texture similar to scrambled eggs. Add soy sauce and turmeric and mix well.

Saute onion and garlic in olive oil. Add tofu, mix and heat.

Makes 2 servings.   3.9 gram net carb each

Quick easy and good!

Entrees

Vegetable Lasagna

½ medium Eggplant	6.3 gram net carb
2 cups Spinach Leaf	0.8 gram net carb
½ pound grated mozzarella	4.9 gram net carb
1 medium Zucchini cut lengthwise into c inch slices	4.4 gram net carb
1 cup Ricotta cheese	8.0 gram net carb
1 Egg	0.4 gram net carb
Pepper to taste	0.4 gram net carb
1 teaspoon Oregano	0.8 gram net carb
¼ teaspoon granulated Garlic	0.4 gram net carb
1 cup low carb spaghetti sauce	6.0 gram net carb
2 tablespoons grated romano	0.8 gram net carb

Preheat oven to 350.

Slice Eggplant into ⅛ inch thick rounds. Mix Ricotta and egg together, ground pepper to taste.

Spread small amount of sauce in bottom of 9x7x2.5 inch baking dish. Add a layer of eggplant slices. Build layers, such as spinach, ½ of mozzarella, zucchini slices, ½ of sauce, eggplant slices, ricotta mixture, spinach, eggplant slices, remaining sauce and mozzarella. Sprinkle spices as you add layers. Cover (with foil) and bake for 90 minutes. Uncover and sprinkle grated Romano over top, bake uncovered another 10–15 minutes.

Makes 6 servings   5.5 gram net carbs each

Yummidy!

Bean Enchiladas

½ cup enchilada sauce	8.0 gram net carb
1 ½ cups shredded cheese (cheddar, Monterey jack)	2.2 gram net carb
¼ cup sour cream	2.0 gram net carb
1 four ounce can green chiles diced	2.9 gram net carb
1 15 ounce can black soy beans	3.5 gram net carb
6 tortillas (low carb)	18 gram net carb

Heat oven to 350.

Combine with one cup of cheese, sour cream, chiles and beans. Stir in ¼ cup enchilada sauce. Salt and pepper to taste.

Lightly oil baking dish and spread small amount of sauce in bottom of dish.

Divide filling equally on the 6 tortillas and roll up. Place seam side down in prepared dish and top with remaining cheese and sauce. Bake until bubbling, approximately 18 minutes.

Makes 6 tortillas   6.1 gram net carbs each using three net carb tortillas

Tastes like more!

Sesame Tofu

2 tablespoons canola oil	0.0 gram net carb
14 ounces firm tofu, drained	5.0 gram net carb
¼ cup sesame seeds	4.2 gram net carb
¼ cup tamari (soy sauce)	3.6 gram net carb

Press the tofu to remove some water. An old bacon press or weighted plate set on tofu will work.

On medium high heat, add oil to skillet.

Slice tofu about ⅜ to ½ inch thick. Dip a slice into bowl containing tamari, covering all sides, then drop into bowl containing sesame seeds, coating completely. Place in hot oiled pan and continue with desired number of pieces. Brown lightly and remove to a paper towel until all are done.

Makes 8 to 10 pieces.   1.3 to 1.6 grams net carbs each

Serve with a side of steamed vegetables.

Chicken Wing Tofu

2 tablespoons canola oil	0.0 gram net carb
14 ounces extra firm tofu, drained	5.0 gram net carb
¼ cup butter	0.0 gram net carb
¼ Frank's Red Hot® sauce or similar	~1.0 gram net carb

Press the tofu to remove some water. An old bacon press or weighted plate set on tofu will work.

On medium high heat, add oil to skillet.

Slice tofu into strips about ⅜ to ½ inch thick. Place in hot oiled pan, brown lightly and remove to a paper towel until all pieces are done.

Melt the butter, add hot sauce and mix.

Dip fried tofu in butter/hot sauce mixture being sure the pieces are completely coated.

Makes 4 servings.   1.5 gram net carbs each

Add or subtract hot sauce to taste.

Southwestern Chili

2 tablespoons chili powder *see note below	1.9 gram net carb
½ teaspoons cumin*	0.8 gram net carb
½ teaspoons oregano*	0.1 gram net carb
¼ large onion	3.3 gram net carb
½ bag (1 1/3 cups) Quorn® grounds	8.0 gram net carb
2 tablespoons olive oil	0.0 gram net carb
2 cloves garlic, minced	1.8 gram net carb
15 ounce can black soy beans	3.5 gram net carb
28 ounce can diced fire roasted tomatoes	30.0 gram net carb
¼ teaspoon salt	0.0 gram net carb
⅛ teaspoon pepper	0.1 gram net carb
crushed red peppers (optional)	
shredded mozzarella or cheddar cheese (optional)	

Heat olive oil in medium size pan over medium high heat. Add onions and garlic; saute. Add Quorn®. Cook until Quorn® is heated through. In separate pan combine drained beans, tomatoes and chili powder. Cook until heated through.

Add Quorn® mixture to beans and tomatoes. Add salt and pepper. Continue to cook for 5 minutes.

Top with crushed red peppers and cheese if you choose.

Makes 6 servings.   8.3g net carbs each

*Some chili powders contain flour. Look for one that does not—or 3 tablespoons of a chili powder containing cumin and oregano.

Simple Broiled Tofu

½ block firm tofu ~½ pound	2.5 gram net carb
2 tablespoons olive oil	0.0 gram net carb
2 tablespoons tamari (soy sauce)	1.8 gram net carb

Preheat oven to broil.

Mix tamari and olive oil.

Cut tofu into ⅜ to ½ inch thick slices. Coat with tamari/oil mixture and place on broiler friendly pan or dish. Broil tofu until lightly browned (~10 minutes) turning often.

Makes 2 servings.   2.2 grams net carb each

Try adding different herbs to the oil for some variety.

Green Pizza

2 low carb tortillas	6.0 gram net carb
2 tablespoons olive oil	0.0 gram net carb
1 tablespoon chopped onion	0.9 gram net carb
½ cup chopped broccoli	1.8 gram net carb
½ small zucchini sliced ¼" thick	1.4 gram net carb
1 cup spinach torn	0.2 gram net carb
2 tablespoons Parmesan cheese	0.4 gram net carb
½ cup mozzarella cheese	1.3 gram net carb
2 tablespoons traditional basil pesto sauce	2.5 gram net carb

Preheat oven to 350.

Heat oil in large skillet. Add onion and saute approximately 4 minutes. Add broccoli and zucchini. Cover and cook until tender. Add spinach and cook for 1 minute. Spread tortillas with pesto. Cover with veggies. Sprinkle with Parmesan cheese and then mozzarella cheese. Bake 7–8 minutes or until cheese is melted.

Makes 8 slices.   1.8 grams net carb each

Absolutely delicious.

Tofu Stirfry

¼ cup canola oil	0.0 gram net carb
¼ teaspoon hot pepper sesame oil(optional)	0.0 gram net carb
14 ounces firm tofu	5.0 gram net carb
4 cups broccoli flowerets	9.9 gram net carb
½ cup mushrooms sliced	0.8 gram net carb
4 scallions (green onions)	2.8 gram net carb
¼ cup tamari (soy sauce)	3.6 gram net carb
¼ cup sliced almonds	1.8 gram net carb
2 cloves garlic, minced	1.8 gram net carb

Press the tofu to remove some water. An old bacon press or weighted plate set on tofu will work. Cut into ½ inch cubes.

On medium high heat, add oil to skillet or wok.

Add minced garlic to heated oil and allow to cook for about thirty seconds or so. Add broccoli and cook to desired texture stirring often. Add tofu, almonds, mushrooms and scallions, stirring until done. Add tamari, stir and serve.

Makes 4 servings.   6.4 grams net carbs each

Great tasting one dish meal.

Tortilla Pizza

2 low carb tortillas	6.0 gram net carb
1 tablespoons olive oil	0.0 gram net carb
½ cup mushrooms sliced	0.8 gram net carb
2 tablespoons lo carb tomato sauce	0.8 gram net carb
¼ teaspoon oregano	0.1 gram net carb
1 tablespoon Parmesan cheese	0.2 gram net carb
½ cup mozzarella cheese	1.3 gram net carb

Preheat oven to 350.

Heat oil in skillet. Add mushrooms and saute until tender. Spread tortillas with tomato sauce and add mushrooms. Sprinkle with Parmesan cheese and then mozzarella cheese. Bake 7–8 minutes or until cheese is melted.

Makes 8 slices.   1.2 grams net carb each

Experiment with toppings but be aware of added carbs.

Tofu in Peanut Sauce

¼ cup Tamari sauce	3.6 gram net carb
1 tablespoon creamy peanut butter	1.3 gram net carb
14 ounces firm tofu, drained	5.0 gram net carb
2 teaspoons vegetable oil	0.0 gram net carb
½ teaspoon hot chili oil	0.0 gram net carb
2 cloves garlic, minced	1.8 gram net carb
1 medium zucchini, cut into strips	4.4 gram net carb
1 medium yellow squash, cut into strips	4.2 gram net carb
2 cups fresh baby spinach leaves	0.8 gram net carb
¼ cup chopped roasted peanuts	2.7 gram net carb

In small bowl whisk tamari sauce into peanut butter. Press tofu with paper towels to remove excess moisture. Cut into ½ inch cubes. Put cubed tofu in baking dish and cover with peanut butter/tamari sauce. Toss with fork to coat. Let set for approx. 20 minutes.

Heat hot chili oil and vegetable oil in large nonstick skillet. Add garlic, zucchini and squash and stir fry for approx. 3 minutes. Add tofu mixture and cook for an additional 2 minutes or until heated through. The sauce will thicken slightly. Stir occasionally.

Stir in spinach and cook until wilted. Sprinkle with chopped nuts.

Makes 5 servings.   4.8 g net carbs each

Yum!

Spinach Souffle

1 10 ounce pkg frozen spinach	3.5 gram net carb
4 eggs	1.6 gram net carb
1 8 ounce package cream cheese	6.2 gram net carb
2 cloves garlic minced	1.8 gram net carb
¼ teaspoon black pepper	0.2 gram net carb
¼ teaspoon salt	0.0 gram net carb
¼ teaspoon tabasco sauce	0.1 gram net carb
2 cups grated Monterey Jack	1.5 gram net carb

Preheated 375 degree oven.

Cook spinach and squeeze dry.
In a large bowl mix spinach, eggs, cream cheese, garlic, salt, pepper and tabasco. Mix well with electric mixer. Add cheese and blend lightly by hand. Lightly oil 8 6oz ramekins and divide mixture between them (or add to 1 quart souffle dish lightly oiled).

Bake at 375 degrees for 30 minutes (ramekins) or 40 minutes (souffle dish).

Makes 8 servings.   1.9 gram net carb each

Good any time of day.

Dave's Beans

2 tablespoons olive oil	0.0 gram net carb
1 clove garlic, sliced	0.9 gram net carb
⅛ onion, sliced	1.6 gram net carb
1 stalk celery sliced diagonally	0.8 gram net carb
¼ cup mushrooms sliced	0.4 gram net carb
14 ounce can black soy beans	3.5 gram net carb
14 ounce can fire roasted diced tomatoes	15.0 gram net carb
2 tablespoons low carb BBQ sauce	~1.0 gram net carb
2 cups raw baby spinach	0.8 gram net carb
½ cup shredded mozzarella cheese	1.2 gram net carb

In large pan heat oil; add garlic, onion, celery and mushrooms. Saute until celery is crisp tender. Stir in soy beans, tomatoes and BBQ sauce. Cook until heated through. Add spinach and cook until wilted. Turn off heat. Sprinkle with mozzarella cheese and cover.

Let sit until cheese is melted.

Makes 4 servings.   6.3 gram net carb each

Spicy and high in protein.

Cajun Tofu

3 green spring onions minced	2.1 gram net carb
2 tablespoons lemon juice	2.0 gram net carb
1 tablespoon olive oil	0.0 gram net carb
2 teaspoons paprika	0.8 gram net carb
½ teaspoon cayenne pepper	0.3 gram net carb
3 cloves garlic, minced	2.7 gram net carb
14–16 ounces firm tofu, drained	5.0 gram net carb

Press tofu to remove excess moisture. Cut into ½ inch cubes. Put cubed tofu in baking dish.

Mix all remaining ingredients and pour over tofu. Toss with fork to coat. Let set for approximately 20 minutes.
Heat large nonstick or lightly oiled skillet. Add tofu mixture and cook until heated through. Stir occasionally.

Double amount of first six ingredients if you want to add sliced zucchini, mushrooms, yellow squash, etc. to marinade.

Makes 4 servings.   3.2 gram net carbs each

Try it on the grill in grilling baskets!

Stuffed Zucchini Italiano

2 medium zucchini	8.8 gram net carb
1 tablespoon butter	0.0 gram net carb
1 cloves garlic, minced	0.9 gram net carb
2 tablespoons chopped onion	1.8 gram net carb
1 cup Sliced Mushrooms	1.5 gram net carb
¾ Cup shredded Mozzarella cheese	1.8 gram net carb
½ cup low carb pasta sauce	3.0 gram net carb
½ teaspoon oregano	0.2 gram net carb
salt and pepper	0.1 gram net carb

Scrub zucchini well, cook whole with a pinch of salt in a pot of boiling water until tender (about 7 to 8 minutes). Preheat oven to 350 degrees. Saute garlic, onion and mushrooms to preference. Cut boiled zucchini in half, lengthwise. Carefully remove squash pulp from skin (shell) with spoon. Chop pulp into small pieces and add to the sauteed ingredients. Salt and pepper to taste. Place shells in oiled baking pan (ie 9x7.5 inch). Add ¼ cup shredded mozzarella and oregano to sauteed ingredients, mix and spoon into shells. Bake, uncovered, 15 minutes. Heat sauce in separate pan. Sprinkle remaining half cup of shredded mozzarella over filled shells and bake for an additional 5 minutes or until cheese is melted. Remove from oven and place shells on plates. Pour heated sauce on top.

Makes 4 pieces.   4.5 g net carbs each

Deelishioso!

Cold Bean and Tempeh Salad

1 15oz can black soy beans	3.5 gram net carb
8 ounces soy tempeh	8.0 gram net carb
2 tablespoons chopped cilantro	0.1 gram net carb
1 large tomato	4.9 gram net carb
¼ cup lime juice	4.0 gram net carb
⅛ teaspoon cayenne	0.1 gram net carb
¼ teaspoon black pepper	0.2 gram net carb

Cut tempeh into ½ inch cubes and steam for about ten minutes.

In a large bowl, mix rinsed beans, cooled tempeh, and remaining ingredients. Place in refrigerator for two hours to overnight stirring occasionally.

Makes 4 servings.   5.2 grams net carb each

Cool.

Veggie Tacos

4 low carb taco shells	12.0 gram net carb
1 tablespoons canola oil	0.0 gram net carb
2 tablespoons chopped onion	1.8 gram net carb
1 small tomato	2.5 gram net carb
Dash cumin, cayenne, oregano, salt	0.1 gram net carb
1 cup Quorn® Grounds	6.0 gram net carb
1 cup shredded green leaf lettuce	0.5 gram net carb
½ cup cheddar cheese	0.7 gram net carb

Preheat oven to 350.

Heat oil in skillet. Add onion and saute until tender. Add Quorn® Grounds and spices, mix and heat.

Put a layer of the cooked and seasoned Quorn® Grounds in taco shell. In layers, add cheese, lettuce and tomato.

Makes 4 tacos.   5.9 grams net carb each

Bueno.

Chicken and Pasta

4 ounces black soy bean pasta	22.0 gram net carb
4 cups raw spinach	1.6 gram net carb
1 13oz can diced vegetarian chicken and gravy	4.0 gram net carb
2 tablespoons olive oil	0.0 gram net carb
¼ teaspoon garlic powder	0.0 gram net carb

Add 4 ounces of black soy bean pasta to boiling water and cook 4 minutes per instructions.

Saute 4 cups of raw spinach in olive oil in large skillet.

Add 2 tablespoons of water to diced chicken and gravy and warm in covered saucepan.

Mix olive oil and garlic in bowl, add drained pasta and toss to coat.

Divide pasta equally onto plates making a hole in the center for equal amounts of spinach. Pour diced chicken and gravy in equal amounts over pasta/spinach.

Salt and pepper to taste.

Makes 4 servings.   6.9 grams net carbs each

Gooood!

Beans and Franks

1 15 ounce can black soy beans	3.5 gram net carb
4 non meat hot dogs	4.0 gram net carb
¼ cup lo carb ketchup	4.0 gram net carb
2 tablespoons lo carb BBQ sauce	2.9 gram net carb
2 tablespoons water	0.0 gram net carb

Slice hot dogs into half inch pieces.

Drain and rinse beans.

Combine all ingredients in a sauce pan, stir and warm on medium heat.

Makes 4 servings.   3.6 grams net carbs each

Quick and tasty!

Side Dishes

Green Salad

2 cups green leaf lettuce   1.0 gram net carb

Use low carb dressings, several brands are available or make a homemade oil and vinegar.

Oil and Vinegar Dressing

⅓ cup wine vinegar   0.0 gram net carb
⅔ cup olive oil   0.0 gram net carb
3 cloves garlic minced   2.8 gram net carb
1 teaspoon black pepper   0.8 gram net carb
½ teaspoon oregano   0.2 gram net carb
1 teaspoon salt   0.0 gram net carb
1 teaspoon basil   0.1 gram net carb

Mix all ingredients in a bowl. Refrigerate for an hour. Stir well before serving.

8 two tablespoon servings   0.5 gram net carb each

Serve with a high protein entree or add protein to salad. Watch the carb count of add ons.

Steamed Vegetables

A simple and nutritious way to prepare a delicious side of vegetables.

Broccoli

1 cup Broccoli   3.5 gram net carb

Cauliflower

1 cup Cauliflower   2.8 gram net carb

Green Beans

1 cup Green Beans   4.2 gram net carb

Asparagus

1 cup Asparagus   2.4 gram net carb

Serve with a high protein entree.

Herbed Oil

¼ cup olive oil	0.0 gram net carb
4 medium mushrooms sliced	0.4 gram net carb
1 teaspoon thyme	0.1 gram net carb
1 pinch salt	0.0 gram net carb
1 pinch black pepper	0.1 gram net carb
1 pinch onion powder	0.1 gram net carb
1 pinch garlic powder	0.1 gram net carb
1 pinch cayenne powder	0.1 gram net carb

Add a tablespoon of the oil to a small saucepan and saute mushrooms. Turn off heat, add remaining oil and dried spices. Stir. Can sit for 1–2 hours to enhance flavors. Heat and use immediately. Replace thyme with rosemary, sage, or a combination to taste.

One serving   0.9 gram net carb each

Use as a topping for low carb pasta, tofu, vegetables, etc..

Spinach Gnocchi

4 oz chopped frozen spinach	1.4 gram net carb
½ lb ricotta cheese	7.5 gram net carb
6 tablespoons grated Parmesan cheese	1.2 gram net carb
salt and freshly ground pepper	0.1 gram net carb
pinch of nutmeg	0.1 gram net carb
1 egg slightly beaten	0.4 gram net carb
3 ½ tablespoons butter	0.0 gram net carb

Thaw spinach and squeeze out moisture. Mix spinach and ricotta cheese, half the Parmesan cheese, salt and pepper and nutmeg. Gradually add egg, beating well.

Use 1 tablespoon of mixture per gnocchi shaping into an oval.

Lower into simmering water 4 at a time cooking gently until gnocchi float to surface (approximately 2 minutes)

Remove with slotted spoon—place in buttered ovenware dish. Repeat the above steps until all are cooked. Sprinkle with remaining Parmesan cheese and dot with butter.

Reheat in 350 degree oven for 10 minutes. Brown under broiler

Makes 4–6 servings   2.6–1.8 gram net carb each

Good!

Broccoli & Cauliflower Salad

½ red bell pepper	2.4 gram net carb
2 cups broccoli	7.0 gram net carb
2 cups cauliflower	5.6 gram net carb
1 tablespoon slivered almonds	1.8 gram net carb
Dressing:	
¼ cup plain unsweetened yogurt	2.9 gram net carb
2 tablespoons lemon juice	1.7 gram net carb
2 tablespoons olive oil	0.0 gram net carb
salt & pepper to taste	0.1 gram net carb
pinch nutmeg	0.1 gram net carb

Slice pepper into matchstick pieces. Trim cauliflower and broccoli into florets. Place in mixing bowl.

Combine dressing ingredients and mix well. Spoon dressing over salad and toss to mix.

Garnish with almond slivers.

Makes 4 servings   5.4 gram net carb each

Serve with a high protein entree.

Zucchini & Onions with Mozzarella

3 tablespoons butter	0.0 gram net carb
3 cups zucchini sliced thinly (⅛").3 medium size	7.8 gram net carb
½ cup (approx. ½ medium onion) 1/8" slices	7.0 gram net carb
½ teaspoon dry basil leaves	0.1 gram net carb
¼ teaspoon dry oregano leaves	0.4 gram net carb
⅛ teaspoon salt	0.0 gram net carb
½ teaspoon minced fresh garlic	0.8 gram net carb
1 cup mozzarella cheese shredded	2.5 gram net carb

In large skillet melt butter, add all ingredients except cheese. Cook stirring frequently until cooked to preferred doneness. Turn off heat, sprinkle with cheese. Put top on pan and let sit for two minutes or until cheese is melted.

Makes 6 servings   3.1 gram net carb each

Yum!

Cheddar Pennies

½ cup butter softened	0.0 gram net carb
1 cup sharp cheddar cheese grated	1.5 gram net carb
1 skinny cup low carb baking mix	0.0 gram net carb
3 tablespoons chopped chives	0.1 gram net carb
¼ teaspoon cayenne pepper	0.1 gram net carb

In large bowl whip butter until creamy, approximately 1 minute. Add grated cheese, bake mix, chives and cayenne pepper. Stir to form a soft ball.

Scrape batter into a log shape on wax paper, forming a long log approximately 1 ½" in diameter. Roll up firmly in wax paper and refrigerate several hours or overnight.

350 degree oven.

Cut dough into slices about ½" thick and bake on greased baking sheets for 12 minutes or until slightly golden.

To get a higher yield, make log a smaller diameter.

Makes approximately 24   0.1 gram net carb each

These are delicious with chili or salad.

Cole Slaw

2 cups shredded white cabbage	4.6 gram net carb
¼ cup shredded red cabbage	0.9 gram net carb
1 teaspoon Dijon mustard	0.2 gram net carb
1 tablespoon apple cider vinegar	0.0 gram net carb
1 teaspoon Splenda®	0.5 gram net carb
⅓ cup mayonnaise	1.6 gram net carb
salt & pepper to taste	0.1 gram net carb

Shred white and red cabbage into large bowl. Add mustard, mayo, vinegar and Splenda®. Mix and, if you'd like, chill in refrigerator.

Serve and salt & pepper to taste.

Makes 4 servings   2.0 gram net carb each

Quick, easy and good.

Pan Roasted Veggies

⅓ cup butter	0.0 gram net carb
½ teaspoon thyme	0.2 gram net carb
¼ teaspoon salt	0.0 gram net carb
¼ teaspoon pepper	0.2 gram net carb
3 cups cauliflower florets	5.1 gram net carb
2 cups broccoli florets	7.4 gram net carb
2 cups green beans	8.3 gram net carb
6 mushrooms sliced	2.0 gram net carb

Place butter in 9 x 13 pan and place 400 degree oven until butter is melted. Add thyme, salt and pepper. Stir. Add veggies and toss to coat with butter. Cover with foil. Bake until crisp tender—approximately 22 minutes.

Makes 6 servings   3.9 gram net carb each

Serve with a high protein entree.

Zucchini with Dill

2 medium zucchini	8.7 gram net carb
1 tablespoon olive oil	0.0 gram net carb
1 tablespoon Parmesan cheese	0.2 gram net carb
1 tablespoon fresh dill chopped	0.1 gram net carb
1 teaspoons red pepper flakes	0.1 gram net carb

Slice the zucchini length wise into strips. Place into boiling water and cook for several minutes until tender but still a bit crisp.

Mix dill, cheese and pepper flakes in small bowl.

Place drained zucchini in a serving bowl, add oil and mix, coating strips. Sprinkle dry mix over zucchini and toss lightly

Makes 2 servings   4.6 gram net carb each

Serve with a high protein entree!

Mashed Cauliflower

4 cups cauliflower florets	6.8 gram net carb
1 tablespoon butter	0.0 gram net carb
1 tablespoon half and half	0.5 gram net carb

Place steamed cauliflower in food processor. Add half & half and butter then puree to preferred consistency.

Makes 4 servings   1.8 gram net carb each

Serve with a high protein entree.

Green Beans

3 tablespoons olive oil	0.0 gram net carb
1 cup sliced mushrooms	1.5 gram net carb
3 cloves garlic minced	2.8 gram net carb
juice of ½ lemon	1.9 gram net carb
½ pound green beans	8.5 gram net carb
¼ cup slivered almonds	2.2 gram net carb

Cut green beans in 3/4" lengths and cook in salted water for 8 minutes.

Heat olive oil in skillet, add mushrooms and saute until brown. Add garlic and lemon juice.
Continue to cook until heated.

Add green beans and sliced almonds. Continue to heat until almonds are warm.

Makes 6 servings   2.8 gram net carb each

Serve with a high protein entree.

Green Beans with Tomatoes

1 pound green beans	17.0 gram net carb
1 cup cherry tomatoes, halved (about 12)	5.3 gram net carb
1 tablespoon shallot, minced	1.7 gram net carb
2 tablespoons olive oil	0.0 gram net carb
2 tablespoons butter	0.0 gram net carb
¼ teaspoon thyme	0.1 gram net carb

In large pan, melt oil and butter over medium high heat. Add thyme and shallot, stir-ring occasionally for 2 minutes. Add green beans and stir occasionally, until beans are crisp tender (5 minutes approx.). Add tomatoes, stir. Cook for approximately a minute.
Serve.

Makes 4–8 servings.   6.0–3.0 gram net carb each

Quick and delicious.

Parmesan Cream Sauce

1 tablespoon butter	0.0 gram net carb
½ cup heavy cream	1.7 gram net carb
¼cup grated parmigiana cheese	0.8 gram net carb
1 small shallot	1.6 gram net carb
¼teaspoon pepper	0.2 gram net carb

Melt butter in a small saucepan on medium heat, add chopped shallot and saute for 2–3 minutes. Add cream and raise heat to boil. Stir in cheese and pepper. As soon as cheese has melted, remove from heat.

Makes 4 servings   1.3 gram net carbs each

Delicious on scrambled eggs or steamed vegetables.

Asparagus Veneto

2 tablespoon olive oil	0.0 gram net carb
1 lb asparagus trimmed	8.1 gram net carb
¼ cup lo carb bread crumbs	4.0 gram net carb
3 tablespoons grated parmigiana cheese	0.6 gram net carb
1 tablespoon parsley	0.0 gram net carb
dash salt	0.0 gram net carb

Preheat oven to 350

Steam asparagus for 4–5 minutes. Place in oven-ready shallow pan.

In small bowl combine bread crumbs, cheese, oil, parsley and salt. Sprinkle on asparagus. Bake 8–10 minutes.

Makes 6 servings   2.1 gram net carbs each

Very good! Serve with a high protein entree.

Mixed Sauteed Vegetables

2 tablespoon olive oil	0.0 gram net carb
1 cup sliced mushrooms	1.5 gram net carb
4 cloves of garlic minced	0.9 gram net carb
½ cup thinly sliced leek	5.5 gram net carb
1 zucchini sliced diagonally	4.4 gram net carb
1 yellow squash sliced diagonally	4.4 gram net carb
¼ red pepper cut into long slivers	1.2 gram net carb
1 teaspoon dried basil	0.3 gram net carb
½ teaspoon rosemary	0.1 gram net carb
½ teaspoon salt	0.0 gram net carb
3 tablespoons grated parmigiana cheese	0.6 gram net carb

Add oil to large skillet on medium heat. When oil is hot add minced garlic. Saute for 2–3 minutes then add remaining vegetables and spices. Continue to cook and mix until desired texture is achieved. Transfer to a serving bowl when done and sprinkle cheese over top.

Makes 6 servings   3.2 gram net carbs each

Very good! Serve with a high protein entree.

Biscuits

1 cup lo carb baking mix	0.0 gram net carb
2 extra large eggs	0.8 gram net carb
2 tablespoons butter softened	0.0 gram net carb
¼ cup water	0.0 gram net carb
⅓ cup oil	0.0 gram net carb

350 degree oven

Combine and mix eggs, water and oil. Add baking mix and stir well. Add softened butter and fold in. Spoon batter in equal portions onto a greased or no stick baking sheet. Sprinkle each biscuit with a ¼ teaspoon of grated Parmesan if desired. 1½ teaspoons of Parmesan totals 0.3 net carb

Bake 12 minutes or until golden brown.

Spread with butter if desired.

Makes 6 very large biscuits   0.2 gram net carb each

Great side for soup, salad or meal! 5.8 grams of protein each.

Black Soy Bean Soup

1 quart (8 cups) water	0.0 gram net carb
1 15 ounce can black soy beans	3.5 gram net carb
¼ cup sliced mushrooms	0.4 gram net carb
2 cloves of garlic minced	0.5 gram net carb
1 small onion	5.9 gram net carb
2 cups chopped broccoli	7.2 gram net carb
6 stalks celery	3.0 gram net carb
2 cups spinach	0.8 gram net carb
¼ teaspoon black pepper	0.2 gram net carb
¼ teaspoon marjoram	0.1 gram net carb
¼ teaspoon rosemary	0.1 gram net carb
½ teaspoon salt	0.0 gram net carb

In a large pot, combine water, garlic, onion, broccoli, celery, spices and salt. Bring to a boil in high heat. Reduce to a simmer and cook for about 45 minutes. Add rinsed beans, mushrooms, and spinach and cook for an additional 15–20 minutes.

Makes 8 servings   2.7 gram net carbs each

Very good!

Celery Cream Soup

2 cups water	0.0 gram net carb
¼ cup sliced onion	2.5 gram net carb
½ teaspoon garlic salt	0.3 gram net carb
2 cups chopped celery	2.4 gram net carb
1 10oz package frozen spinach	3.5 gram net carb
1 cup cottage cheese	6.0 gram net carb
⅛ teaspoon black pepper	0.1 gram net carb
½ cup sour cream	4.9 gram net carb
2 cups low carb milk	6.0 gram net carb

In a large pot, combine water, onion, celery, and spinach. Bring to a boil, cover reduce heat and simmer until vegetables are tender (about 12–15 minutes). When done transfer to a blender, add cottage cheese and blend until smooth. Return to pot, add milk and spices, and reheat. Serve with grated cheddar or Romano on top if desired.

Makes 8 servings   3.2 gram net carbs each

Easy and good!

Desserts

Chocolate Almond Cheesecake

½ cups Splenda®	12.0 gram net carb
1 tablespoon liquid stevia extract	0.0 gram net carb
4 eight ounce pkgs cream cheese softened	32.0 gram net carb
4 extra large eggs	1.8 gram net carb
1 cup sour cream	8.0 gram net carb
1 tablespoon unsweetened cocoa	1.1 gram net carb
2 teaspoons vanilla extract	0.0 gram net carb
1 teaspoon almond extract	0.0 gram net carb
1 cup low carb chocolate chips melted	11.2 gram net carb
⅔ cup almonds finely chopped	4.6 gram net carb

325 degree oven

In large mixer bowl beat Splenda® and cream cheese until light and fluffy. Continue beating adding eggs one at a time until creamy. Add remaining ingredients except chocolate chips and almonds. Continue beating until well mixed.

By hand fold in melted chocolate to swirl throughout batter for a marbled effect. Lightly butter a 9" springform pan. Press chopped almonds firmly into bottom of pan. Pour batter into prepared pan.

Bake 70 minutes. Turn off oven and leave cheesecake in oven for 2 hours. Loosen sides of cheesecake from pan by running a knife around inside of pan. Let cool completely. Cover and refrigerate overnight or 8 hours.

Makes 16 servings   4.4 gram net carbs per serving

Absolutely tastes like more!

Whipped Cream

½ cup heavy whipping cream   3.3 gram net carb
8 drops vanilla   0.0 gram net carb
4 drops Stevia   0.0 gram net carb

Cool bowl and beaters in refrigerator.

Combine ingredients in bowl. Beat on high speed until desired texture is obtained (4–5 minutes). Over mixing will turn cream into butter.

4-¼cup servings.   0.8 gram net carb each

A nice topping can enhance desserts.

Walnut Chocolate Chip Cookies

½ cup MiniCarb® baking mix	0.0 gram net carb
½ cup ground walnuts	2.8 gram net carb
¼ cup Splenda®	6.0 gram net carb
1 teaspoon liquid stevia extract	0.0 gram net carb
1 stick butter (½ cup), room temperature	0.0 gram net carb
1 extra large egg	0.5 gram net carb
2 tablespoons water	0.0 gram net carb
or low carb milk, soy milk	Varies
1 teaspoon vanilla extract	0.0 gram net carb
¼ cup low carb® chocolate chips	3.2 gram net carb

325 degree oven

Combine bake mix, splenda and ground walnuts in bowl. Add butter and beat in. Mix egg, water, stevia and vanilla and add to bake mix. Mix thoroughly. Stir in chocolate chips.

Divide batter equally on cookie sheet. Bake 15 minutes.

Makes 12 cookies   1.0 gram net carb each

Who says you can't have cookies every day.

Chocolate Hazelnut Bars

Crust

½ cup hazelnuts	4.7 gram net carb
¾ cup MiniCarb® bake mix	0.0 gram net carb
¼ cup Splenda®	6.0 gram net carb
6 tablespoons cold butter cut into pieces	0.0 gram net carb

Chocolate Topping

¼ cup Splenda®	6.0 gram net carb
2 teaspoons stevia	0.0 gram net carb
⅓ cup unsweetened cocoa powder	6.0 gram net carb
2 tablespoons butter	0.0 gram net carb
⅓ cup water	0.0 gram net carb
2 extra large eggs	0.8 gram net carb
1 ½ teaspoons vanilla extract	0.0 gram net carb

350 degree oven
Bake hazelnuts on baking sheet in oven for 7 minutes. Remove and cool.
Lightly oil 8" square baking pan.

In food processor with metal blade grind hazelnuts with MiniCarb® bake mix and Splenda until it looks like fine crumbs. Add butter pieces and using a pulse action process until coarse crumbs form. Pour mixture into oiled pan and press out evenly. Bake 22 minutes. Remove from oven and let cool.

In medium saucepan stir together Splenda® and cocoa powder. Gradually whisk in water until it is smooth. Over medium heat cook until Splenda dissolves. Remove from heat. Stir in butter until melted. Beat in eggs and vanilla extract. Pour over baked crust.

Bake 20 minutes or until topping is set. Remove and let cool completely.
Cut into 2 inch bars.

Makes 16 bars   1.5 gram net carb each

Nice treat.

Chocolate Brownies

3 ounces unsweetened chocolate	11.0 gram net carb
½ cup butter	0.0 gram net carb
½ cup Splenda	12.0 gram net carb
2 teaspoon Stevia Liquid Extract	0.0 gram net carb
3 extra large eggs	1.2 gram net carb
¼ cup vegetable oil	0.0 gram net carb
1 teaspoon vanilla extract	0.0 gram net carb
½ cup chopped (coarsely) walnuts	4.1 gram net carb
1 cup MiniCarb® bake mix	0.0 gram net carb

Chocolate glaze

½ cup dark chocolate sugar free chips	5.6 gram net carb
2 tablespoons water	0.0 gram net carb
or low carb milk or soy milk	Varies
2 tablespoons butter	0.0 gram net carb
1 teaspoon vanilla extract	0.0 gram net carb

325 degree oven

Lightly oil 9 x 13" baking pan. In medium size saucepan melt chocolate and butter on low heat until smooth and completely melted. Remove from heat. Stir in Splenda until blended well. Add eggs one at a time, beating well after each addition. Add nuts, stevia, oil and vanilla extract. Beat again. Add bake mix and stir until blended. Batter will be stiff. Spread in baking pan.
Bake approximately 20 minutes or until toothpick comes out of center with crumbs. Do not over bake. Remove from oven and cool.

To make glaze, melt chocolate chips with butter. Stir in water until smooth. Remove from heat and add vanilla. Stir. Spread on brownies and decorate with walnut halves if desired.

Makes 12 brownies. 2.8 gram net carb each

Yum!

Walnut Spice Cookies

½ cup MiniCarb® baking mix	0.0 gram net carb
½ cup ground walnuts	2.8 gram net carb
¼ cup Splenda®	6.0 gram net carb
1 teaspoon liquid stevia extract	0.0 gram net carb
1 teaspoon cinnamon	0.6 gram net carb
1 stick (½ cup) butter room temperature	0.0 gram net carb
1 large egg	0.4 gram net carb
2 tablespoons water	0.0 gram net carb
1 teaspoon vanilla extract	0.0 gram net carb

Combine dry ingredients in large bowl. Mix butter, egg, stevia, water and vanilla. Add to dry ingredients and stir well.

325 degree oven.

Divide batter equally on the cooking sheet. Bake for 15 minutes.

Makes 12 cookies.   0.8 gram net carb each

Spicy and sweet!

Thumb Print Cookies

½ cup MiniCarb® bake mix	0.0 gram net carb
1 teaspoon Stevia liquid extract	0.0 gram net carb
¼ cup butter softened	0.0 gram net carb
1 teaspoon vanilla extract	0.0 gram net carb
1 extra large egg	0.4 gram net carb
¼ cup water	0.0 gram net carb
5 tablespoons low carb jam	10.0 gram net carb

Preheated 325 degree oven

Mix egg, stevia, water, butter and vanilla, beating well. Stir in bake mix until well blended.

Between your hands, lightly roll tablespoonful size amounts of wet batter and place on ungreased baking sheet about 3 inches apart. Dent surface of batter rounds with wet thumb. Bake 12 minutes and remove pan from oven. Add teaspoon amounts of low carb jam to the depression. Return to oven and continue to bake another 3–4 minutes.

Makes 15 cookies   0.7 gram net carb each

Great snack!

Strawberry Torte

Crust:

1 cup no carb bake mix	0.0 gram net carb
2 extra large eggs	0.8 gram net carb
4 tablespoons butter softened	0.0 gram net carb
⅔ cup heavy cream	4.4 gram net carb
½ teaspoon vanilla extract	0.0 gram net carb
3 tablespoons Splenda	4.5 gram net carb
⅓ cup oil	0.0 gram net carb

Combine above ingredients and spread on a round 12" baking sheet. Bake 350 degrees for 20 minutes.

While baking the crust, in medium bowl combine

8 ounces cream cheese slightly softened	6.2 gram net carb
½ cup ricotta cheese	3.7 gram net carb
¼ cup Splenda	8.0 gram net carb
2 teaspoons vanilla extract	0.0 gram net carb

Remove crust from oven and spread the cream cheese mixture evenly over it. Bake for 4 minutes.

Remove from oven and sprinkle with

2 cups sliced strawberries	18.9 gram net carb
Makes 12 servings	3.9 carbs per serving

Decadent!!!

Coconut Almond Cookies

½ cup MiniCarb® baking mix	0.0 gram net carb
½ cup toasted coconut	2.5 gram net carb
¼ cup Splenda®	6.0 gram net carb
1 teaspoon liquid stevia extract	0.0 gram net carb
1 teaspoon almond extract	0.0 gram net carb
1 stick (½ cup) butter room temperature	0.0 gram net carb
1 large egg	0.4 gram net carb
2 tablespoons water	0.0 gram net carb
1 teaspoon vanilla extract	0.0 gram net carb

Combine dry ingredients in large bowl. Mix butter, egg, stevia, water, almond extract and vanilla. Stir well.

325 degree oven.
Divide batter equally on the cooking sheet. Bake for 15 minutes.

Makes 12 cookies. 0.7 gram net carb each

Tasty combination of flavors.

Vanilla Ice Cream and Peanut Butter

½ cup low carb vanilla ice cream   3.0 gram net carb
1 tablespoon peanut butter   1.3 gram net carb
1 tablespoon low carb chocolate chips   0.4 gram net carb

Press the ice cream into a 6 ounce custard cup leaving a depression in the center with the ice cream thickness approximately the same on the sides and the bottom
Drop the peanut butter into the depression and sprinkle the chocolate chips over the ice cream and peanut butter.

1 serving.   4.7 gram net carb each

Quick, simple, delicious!

Coconut Pine Nut Cookies

½ cup MiniCarb® baking mix	0.0 gram net carb
¼ cup coconut	1.3 gram net carb
¼ cup pine nuts	3.2 gram net carb
¼ cup Splenda®	6.0 gram net carb
1 teaspoon liquid stevia extract	0.0 gram net carb
1 teaspoon almond extract	0.0 gram net carb
1 stick (½ cup) butter room temperature	0.0 gram net carb
1 large egg	0.4 gram net carb
2 tablespoons water	0.0 gram net carb
1 teaspoon vanilla extract	0.0 gram net carb

Combine dry ingredients in large bowl. Mix butter, egg, stevia, water, almond extract and vanilla. Stir well.

325 degree oven.

Divide batter equally on the cooking sheet. Bake for 15 minutes.

Makes 12 cookies.   0.9 gram net carb each

Gooood!

Almond Cookies

½ cup no carb baking mix	0.0 gram net carb
¼ cup sliced almonds	1.8gram net carb
¼ cup almond butter	5.1 gram net carb
¼ cup Splenda®	6.0 gram net carb
1 teaspoon liquid stevia extract	0.0 gram net carb
1 teaspoon almond extract	0.0 gram net carb
1 stick (½ cup) butter room temperature	0.0 gram net carb
1 large egg	0.4 gram net carb
2 tablespoons water	0.0 gram net carb
1 teaspoon vanilla extract	0.0 gram net carb

Combine dry ingredients in large bowl. Mix butter, egg, stevia, water, almond extract and vanilla. Stir well.
325 degree oven.

Divide batter equally on the cooking sheet. Bake for 15 minutes.

Makes 12 cookies.   1.1 gram net carb each

Almondy!

Chocolate Walnut Squares

1 cup no carb bake mix	0.0 gram net carb
½ cup Splenda®	12.0 gram net carb
2 teaspoons liquid stevia extract	0.0 gram net carb
1 teaspoon cinnamon	0.6 gram net carb
2 extra large eggs	0.8 gram net carb
¾ cup water	0.0 gram net carb
1 cup walnuts, coarsely chopped	8.4 gram net carb
2 tablespoons vanilla extract	0.0 gram net carb
2 tablespoons butter, room temperature	0.0 gram net carb
2 one ounce squares unsweetened baking chocolate	7.7 gram net carb
1 tablespoon butter	0.0 gram net carb
2 tablespoons half and half	1.3 gram net carb

Preheat oven to 325.

In large bowl combine water, eggs, vanilla, stevia and butter. Add bake mix, Splenda®, cinnamon and walnuts and stir until well blended.
In small pan on low heat, melt chocolate and butter, stirring constantly. Stir in half and half. Pour chocolate mixture over batter and softly fold in.

Pour batter into buttered 8 x 8 square pan.

Bake for 20 minutes.

Let cool and cut into squares.

Makes 16 squares.   1.9 gram net carb each

Absolutely delicious.

Hot Chocolate Cupcakes

1½ teaspoons no carb bake mix	0.0 gram net carb
3 teaspoons Splenda®	4.5 gram net carb
1 extra large eggs	0.8 gram net carb
1 egg yolk	0.6 gram net carb
½ teaspoon vanilla extract	0.0 gram net carb
3 tablespoons butter	0.0 gram net carb
1 one ounce square unsweetened baking chocolate	3.9 gram net carb

Preheat oven to 375.

Coat the inside of 2 6 oz ramekins, souffle dishes or pyrex custard cups with butter. Dust the inside of dishes with baking mix, shaking out excess.

In small pan on low heat, melt chocolate and butter, stirring as needed.

In a medium bowl, mix egg, egg yolk, Splenda®, and vanilla using a high speed mixer until it just peaks when mixer is pulled out.

Remove chocolate from heat. Allow to cool slightly and stir in bake mix. Slowly pour chocolate mixture over egg mixture and softly fold in.

Divide batter into the buttered cups.

Place cups on baking pan and bake for 9 minutes.

Let cool slightly and turn out on to plate using a knife around the inside of cup.

Makes 2 servings.   4.9 gram net carb each

Add a dollop of whipped cream or a side of vanilla ice cream.

Strawberry Shorts Cake

Cake

½ cup MiniCarb® bake mix	0.0 gram net carb
1 teaspoon Stevia liquid extract	0.0 gram net carb
¼ cup butter softened	0.0 gram net carb
1 teaspoon vanilla extract	0.0 gram net carb
1 extra large egg	0.4 gram net carb
¼ cup water	0.0 gram net carb

Filling

1 cup sliced strawberries	9.5 gram net carb
1 teaspoon Stevia liquid extract	0.0 gram net carb
¼ cup water	0.0 gram net carb

325 degree oven

Mix one teaspoon of Stevia in one quarter cup of water and pour over the sliced strawberries. Allowing to sit will blend the flavors and sweetness.

Mix egg, stevia, water, butter and vanilla, beating well. Stir in bake mix until well blended.

Using a spatula, smear the insides of four lightly buttered, oven proof, six ounce ramekins (or custard cups) with batter. A thin coat over the entire inside of the cups will use all of the batter. Put cups on cookie sheet or similar and place in preheated oven. Bake for 20 minutes. Allow to cool. Cakes should easily pop out of cup. Spoon in strawberry mixture and add a dollop of whipped cream (adds approximately 0.8 net carb per quarter cup).

Makes 4 cakes   2.5 grams net carb each

Yummmmmmmm!

Root Beer Float

½ cup low carb vanilla ice cream   3.0 gram net carb
8–12 ounces no carb root beer   0.0 gram net carb

Place scoop of ice cream in a tall glass. Add root beer to cause foaming. Eat with spoon and drink with straw. Mix as desired.

1 serving.   3.0 gram net carb each

Cool and fun.

Peanut Butter Swirl Cake

cake:

1½ cup no carb bake mix	0.0 gram net carb
¼ cup Splenda®	6.0 gram net carb
2 teaspoons liquid stevia extract	0.0 gram net carb
2 extra large eggs	0.8 gram net carb
1 cup water	0.0 gram net carb
¼ cup smooth peanut butter	5.0 gram net carb
1 tablespoons vanilla extract	0.0 gram net carb
¼ canola oil	0.0 gram net carb
1 tablespoon butter	0.0 gram net carb
1 one ounce squares unsweetened baking chocolate	3.9 gram net carb
¼ cup smooth peanut butter	5.0 gram net carb

frosting:

⅓ cup smooth peanut butter	3.5 gram net carb
⅓ cup Splenda®	8.0 gram net carb
1 teaspoons liquid stevia extract	0.0 gram net carb
¼ cup half and half	2.6 gram net carb

Preheat oven to 325.

In large bowl combine water, eggs, vanilla, stevia, peanut butter and oil. Add bake mix, Splenda®, and stir until well blended.

In small pan on low heat, melt chocolate and butter, stirring in peanut butter once melted. Pour chocolate/PB mixture over batter and softly fold in. Pour batter into a no stick or buttered cake pan. Bake for 20 minutes.

Mix frosting ingredients in bowl and cover cooled or slightly warm cake.

Makes 12 servings.   2.9 gram net carb each

Absolutely delicious.

Carb Counter

Food	Portion	Grams Total Carb	Grams Net Carb
Grains			
Barley pearled cooked	1 cup	44.3	38.3
Buckwheat rsted cooked	1 cup	33.5	29.0
Bulgur cooked	1 cup	33.8	25.6
Couscous cooked	1 cup	36.5	34.3
Rice, brown cooked	1 cup	36.4	34.2
Rice, instant cooked	1 cup	35.1	34.1
Millet cooked	1 cup	41.2	38.9
Cornmeal yellow whole	1 cup	93.8	84.9
Cereal			
Oatmeal cooked	1.25 cup	25.3	21.3
Puffed Wheat	1 cup	11.9	10.1
Shredded Wheat	2 biscuits	36.2	30.7
Muesli fruit & nut	1 cup	66.1	59.9
Rice Chex	1 cup	21.3	21.1
All Bran	⅓ cup	24.0	11.1
Corn Flakes	1 cup	24.2	23.4
Cheerios	1 cup	22.2	18.6
Cream of Wheat cooked	1 cup	25.2	21.2
Special K	1 cup	22.0	21.3
Rice Crispies	1 cup	22.8	22.5
Life	¾ cup	25.0	22.9
Breads			
Blueberry Muffins (113g)	Medium	54.2	51.3
Bagel plain	4½ inch	70.0	67.0
Pumpernickel	Slice	12.4	10.7
White	Slice	12.7	12.1
Rye	Slice	15.5	13.6
Pita Whole Wheat	6.5 inch	35.2	30.5
English Muffin	1	26.2	24.7

Food	Portion	Grams Total Carb	Grams Net Carb
Crackers			
Graham	1 rectangle	5.4	5.2
Saltine	1 rectangle	4.3	4.1
Rice cakes brown rice	1	7.3	6.9
Wheat thins	1 serving	20.0	19.1
Pasta			
Whole Wheat cooked	1 cup	37.2	30.9
Spaghetti cooked	1 cup	39.7	37.3
Corn Pasta cooked	1 cup	39.1	32.4
Rice Pasta	1 cup	43.3	38.3
Beans			
Black Turtle cooked	1 cup	40.8	25.8
Garbanzo cooked	1 cup	45.0	32.5
Lentils cooked	1 cup	39.9	24.3
Kidney cooked	1 cup	40.4	29.1
Lima cooked	1 cup	39.3	26.1
Pinto cooked	1 cup	44.8	29.4
Soy cooked	1 cup	17.1	6.8
Edamame cooked	1 cup	19.3	12.3
Black Soy canned	1 cup	16.0	2.0
Nuts			
Almonds sliced	1 cup	18.2	7.3
Cashews dry rstd halves	1 cup	44.8	40.7
Peanuts dry roasted	1 cup	31.4	19.7
Walnuts chopped	1 cup	16.0	8.2

Food	Portion	Grams Total Carb	Grams Net Carb
Fruit			
Apple slices	1 cup	15.2	12.6
Apricot slices	1 cup	18.4	15.1
Banana sliced	1 cup	34.3	30.4
Blueberries	1 cup	21.0	17.5
Cantaloupe cubes	1 cup	13.1	11.7
Cherries sweet pitted	1 cup	23.2	20.2
DateDeglet nopit chopped	1 cup	133.6	119.4
Fig raw large	1	12.3	10.4
Grapefruit white sections	1 cup	19.3	16.8
Grapes red/white seedless	1 cup	29.0	27.6
Kiwi	1 cup	26.0	20.7
Mango slices	1 cup	28.1	25.1
Orange sections	1 cup	21.2	16.9
Papaya cubes	1 cup	13.7	11.2
Peach slices	1 cup	16.2	13.7
Pear slices	1 cup	25.5	20.4
Pineapple diced	1 cup	19.6	17.4
Plum sliced	1 cup	18.8	16.5
Raisins seedless packed	1 cup	130.7	124.6
Raspberry	1 cup	14.7	6.7
Strawberries sliced	1 cup	12.8	9.5
Watermelon diced	1 cup	11.5	10.9
Dairy			
Butter	1 cup	0.1	0.1
Half & Half	1 cup	10.4	10.4
Cream Heavy	1 cup	6.6	6.6
Cheddar Cheese shredded	1 cup	1.5	1.5
Monterey Jack shredded	1 cup	0.8	0.8
Mozzarella shredded	1 cup	2.5	2.5
Cream Cheese	1 cup	6.2	6.2
Egg extra large	1	0.4	0.4

Food	Portion	Grams Total Carb	Grams Net Carb
Meat Substitutes			
Quorn Grounds	⅔ Cup	5.0	1.0
Quorn Cutlet	1 cutlet	20.0	16.0
Quorn Pattie	1 pattie	12.0	9.0
Quorn Turkey Roast	1/5roast 90g	8.0	2.0
Boca Burger	1 burger	5.0	1.0
Lightlife Smart Dog	1 dog	2.0	1.0
Ltlife Sausage Grounds	2 oz	4.0	2.0
Lightlife Ground Beef	2 oz	4.0	2.0
Lightlife Deli Ham	4 slices	5.0	4.0
Lightlife Deli Turkey	4 slices	4.0	3.0
Lightlife Deli Bologna	4 slices	2.0	0.0
Tofu Extra Firm WaterPk	3 oz	2.0	1.0
White Wave Seitan	85 grams	3.0	2.0
Tempeh	4 oz	14.0	4.0
Pasta			
Whole Wheat cooked	1 cup	37.2	30.9
Spaghetti cooked	1 cup	39.7	37.3
Corn Pasta cooked	1 cup	39.1	32.4
Rice Pasta cooked	1 cup	43.3	38.0

Food	Portion	Grams Total Carb	Grams Net Carb
Vegetables			
Asparagus cooked	1 cup	5.2	2.4
Broccoli cooked chopped	1 cup	11.0	6.0
Cabbage raw shredded	1 cup	3.9	2.3
Cauliflower raw	1 cup	5.3	2.8
Celery raw chopped	1 cup	3.0	1.4
Cucumber slices	1 cup	3.8	3.5
Eggplant cooked	1 cup	8.6	6.1
Green Beans cooked	1 cup	9.9	5.9
Lettuce green leaf shred	1 cup	1.0	0.5
Mushroom slices	1 cup	2.3	1.5
Onion raw slices	1 cup	11.6	10.0
Peppers green sweet chop	1 cup	6.9	4.4
Spinach raw	1 cup	1.1	0.4
Zucchini raw sliced	1 cup	3.8	2.6
Beets cooked	1 cup	16.9	13.5
Raw Carrot grated	1 cup	10.5	7.4
Cooked Carrots slices	1 cup	12.8	8.2
Green Peas raw	1 cup	21.0	13.6
GreenPeas edible pod raw	1 cup	4.8	3.2
Potato baked no skin	1 cup	13.2	12.3
Tomato 3" diameter ripe	1	7.1	4.9
Corn cooked no cob	1 cup	31.7	27.7
Sweet Potato mashed	1 cup	58.1	49.9
French Fries (in oil)	3.5 ounces	39.8	36.3

Food	Portion	Grams Total Carb	Grams Net Carb
Drinks			
Apple Juice unsweetened	1 cup	29.0	28.8
Beer regular	12 oz	10.75	10.75
Carrot Juice canned	1 cup	21.9	20.0
Cola regular	12 oz	39.8	39.8
Milk 2%	1 cup	11.4	11.4
Skim Milk	1 cup	12.2	12.2
Orange Juice Fresh	1 cup	25.8	25.3
Pineapple Juice canned	1 cup	34.5	34.5
Herbal Tea	6 oz	0.4	0.4
Sweeteners			
Sugar granulated	1 cup	200.0	200.0
Brown sugar packed	1 cup	214.0	214.1
Stevia liquid glycerite	1 tbsp	0.0	0.0
Splenda® granular	1 cup	24.0	24.0
Molasses	1 cup	251.8	251.8
Flours			
All purpose White Flour	1 cup	95.4	92.0
Whole Wheat Flour	1 cup	87.1	72.5
Brown Rice Flour	1 cup	120.8	113.5
Flax Seed	1 cup	53.1	9.9
Soy Flour	1 cup	29.6	21.5

INDEX

chicken wing tofu, 54
chile, southwestern, 27
chocolate almond cheesecake, 88
chocolate brownies, 92
chocolate chip cookies, walnut, 90
chocolate chips, 24, 26, 40, 88, 90, 92, 97
chocolate cupcakes, hot, 101
chocolate hazelnut bars, 91
chocolate walnut squares, 100
cholesterol, 1, 9-13, 18-19, 22-23
cholesterol content in food, 12
chromium, 21
cigarette, 13
cream, 5, 8, 12, 23-24, 26-30, 35-38, 40-41, 44-45, 47, 49, 52, 61, 82, 87-89, 95, 97, 101-103
cream, whipped, 47
cocaine, 15
coconut almond cookies, 96
coconut pine nut cookies, 98
cold bean and tempeh salad, 65
cole slaw, 76
complex carbs, 15
composure, 21
concentration, 16
cookies, 15, 24, 27, 90, 93-94, 96, 98-99
cookies,
    almond, 99
    coconut almond, 46, 96
    coconut pine nut, 98
    thumb print, 94
    walnut chocolate chip, 90
    walnut spice, 27, 93
Cortisol, 13
craving, 10, 15-16
C Reactive Protein, CRP, 9, 10, 17
dairy, 12
depression, 1, 11, 13, 18-19, 22, 94, 97
diabetes, 0-1, 9, 11, 13, 15, 18
diarrhea, 20

diastolic, 17
digestive tract, 14
dinner, 16, 26-27
Disability, 18
dressing, oil and vinegar, 69
Eden®, 24
Egg Beaters®, 12, 23, 28
eggs, 4, 12, 28-31, 33-34, 36, 38, 41, 44-45, 48-50, 61, 82, 85, 88, 91-92, 95, 100-101, 104
    baked, 7, 24-25, 27, 36, 43, 91
    scrambled eggs with bread cubes, 31
    scrambled eggs with asparagus, 49
    shirred, 48
emotional healing, 20
enchiladas, bean, 52
energy, 0-1, 3-4, 11, 15-16, 18, 21
essential fatty acids, 22
excess insulin, 10-12, 15-16
exercise, 0, 19
fat, 1, 3-4, 8-11, 13-16, 19, 21, 24-25, 28
fat burning, 3, 11, 25
fat cells, 9, 13
fat storing, 4, 10-11, 16
fatigue, 11
feet, 11
fiber, 3-4, 15, 20, 23
fibromyalgia, 18
flaxseed, 22
float, root beer, 103
french toast, 27, 38
frittata,
    spinach, 33
    zucchini mushroom, 34
fructose, 3, 10
gas, 14, 20
glucose, 3-5, 9-11, 13, 17, 19-21
glycation chemistry, 10
glycerin, 20
Glycemic Index, 4-5, 25, 28

sugar, 2-4, 9-11, 13, 15-17, 20-22, 24-25, 92

sugar alcohols, 20-21, 24

Sympathetic Nervous System, 13

sympathetic response, 19

systolic, 17

tacos, veggie, 66

target heart rate, 19

thyroid, 22

toast, 4, 15, 16, 26, 27, 36, 48

tobacco, 15

tofu,
  broiled, 56
  cajun, 63
  chicken wing, 54
  in peanut sauce, 60
  scramble, 41, 50
  sesame, 27, 53, 58
  stirfry, 58

torte, strawberry, 95

tortilla, 23, 27, 41, 59

triglycerides, 1, 17-19

turkey, 23-24

Tyrosine, 22

ulcers, 1, 14, 18

vanilla ice cream and peanut butter, 97

vegetable lasagna, 26, 51

vegetables, mixed sauteed, 84

vegetables, steamed, 70

vegetarians, 2, 10, 21

veggie tacos, 66

veggies, pan roasted, 77

Vitamin B12, 21

Vitamin B complex, 21, 22

Vitamin C, 21

Vitamin D, 12

Vitamin E, 21

walking, 19

walnut chocolate chip cookies, 90

walnut spice cookies, 27, 93

walnut squares, chocolate, 100

water, 23, 25

weakness, 16, 20

weight, 1-2, 9, 11, 13, 15, 17, 19, 22

weight loss, 2, 9, 19

well being, 19, 22

whipped cream, 89

White Wave, 24

Worthington®, 24

Yoga, 20

Yves®, 24

zucchini with dill, 78

zucchini & onions with mozzarella, 74

978-0-595-35985-1
0-595-35985-X

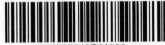

Made in the USA
Lexington, KY
24 February 2012